WELCOME
TO MY
COUNTRY

WELCOME TO MY COUNTRY

LAUREN SLATER

HAMISH HAMILTON · LONDON

HAMISH HAMILTON LTD
Published by the Penguin Group
Penguin Books Ltd, 27 Wrights Lane, London W8 5TZ, England
Penguin Books USA Inc., 375 Hudson Street, New York, New York 10014, USA
Penguin Books Australia Ltd, Ringwood, Victoria, Australia
Penguin Books Canada Ltd, 10 Alcorn Avenue, Toronto, Ontario, Canada M4V 3B2
Penguin Books (NZ) Ltd, 182-190 Wairau Road, Auckland 10, New Zealand
Penguin Books Ltd, Registered Offices: Harmondsworth, Middlesex, England

First published in the United States of America by Random House 1996
First published in Great Britain by Hamish Hamilton Ltd 1996
1 3 5 7 9 10 8 6 4 2

Portions of this work were originally published in
Creative Nonfiction, *Missouri Review*, and *New Letters* magazine.
'Striptease' appeared in *Best American Essays, 1994*

Typeset in Sabon
Printed in Great Britain by Clays Ltd, St Ives plc

A CIP catalogue for this book is available from the British Library
ISBN 0-241-13638-5

The tales related in this book are based on my true experience with real patients whom I have treated. However, in every case the patient's name, physical characteristics, and specific biographical details have been altered so as to protect and respect the confidentiality of all involved. All involved have approved their disguises. In a few cases, the individuals represented are complete composite portraits, made up of many different images and from the many different stories I have heard in my practice as a psychologist. My aim has been to remain true to the subjective experience of mental illness as I have perceived it, while at the same time honoring the ethic of privacy inherent in any doctor/patient relationship.

In all cases where the story is based on an individual patient, however loosely (as opposed to a complete composite portrait), I have obtained written consent from the individual involved. In all cases, patients were eager to have aspects of their suffering, however disguised the form, shared with the wider world in the hopes that others might come to a better understanding of their plight.

For my seven sisters

PREFACE

Alfred Adler, one of the leading psychiatrists of the twentieth century, used to say that people's earliest memories stand as a symbol for the conflicts that bring them to treatment. According to Adler, if you recall being on a beach at two years of age, walking close to the tarry tide and seeing a dead seagull with its eyes still startled open, then the work of therapy should begin here, with the experience of death and how it rises in you. Or if you recall the garage where your father worked, the smell of oil and silvery teeth of a saw, then this is where you must begin, unraveling the knots of violence that simmer between parent and child.

Where, I have often wondered, am I? I go back, winding through the gray canals of my brain, pause at the dollhouse, where the windows were as small as my milk teeth and a plastic baby slept in a cradle, its mouth a splash of red. Here? No, not here, back still farther, to a housekeeper with wiry hair and cake batter dripping from the wooden spoon she held. *Open up,* she said, and sugar sang through me. What a lovely place to start. But no, not here. Drop lower. And it is summertime, a season I have always hated, and trees wilt in the windless air. Here. Here. A cat cries high up on the hill next to our house. Air conditioners drip and weep, darkening the parched gardens beneath them, and if I press my feet to the ground I can almost feel the roots sucking up the moisture, the crimson cups of poppies asking for more. My sister, blond and dressed in frills, comes out the door, takes my hand, and leads me down the silent street. I don't know language yet, and so the only words I hear are the mixed-up alphabets of birds and motors, murmurs and scary shrieks. This is the world of the child.

And my sister leads me down the street. She is two years older than I and possessed of wonderful talents: the talent of talk, of balanced walk, of drinking gracefully from glass cups. I think she is singing to me, but when I look up at her face I can't connect the movement of her lips with the melody in the air. Her lips open, and moments later notes float into my consciousness, as if I were seeing a movie where voice and action weren't synchronized. And even though I'm only two or so, a feeling of separateness comes over me, a knowledge of the rifts between music and its maker, between sun and what it strikes, between her hand and mine, which are woven together but which suddenly I can't really feel.

She stops, bends over, grasps a flower growing behind a neighbor's fence. Perhaps it was a lady's slipper or a mandrake, white with lanky tendrils, each one knobbed at the tip. She buries her face in the plenitude and then stretches the stem toward me. *Here. Smell.* But I can't. The heat clutches at me. The sky doesn't make sense. I try to smell but suddenly my nose is a closed canal and the world grows gray and tiny. The flower appears as if from a great distance, stiff and artificial, utterly devoid of comfort. *Here. Smell.* The stem shrieks; the petals are dead wax. This is what it means to lose the world, moments when the cord between you and someone else withers.

"Yes," Adler might say. "So your search has been one of connection, an attempt to repair the rifts between yourself and others." Yes, I would respond, and while I recognize that as a central struggle for all humankind, I believe, for a variety of reasons that have to do with my own life, that I am particularly sensitive to those rifts because they come to me as disembodied states, extreme dissociations.

So. My search, and the searches of separate others, represented here in episodes from my work as a psychologist. My patients—borderline personalities, sociopaths, bulimics, schizophrenics of every type— are foreign, tropical, green roses and striped plants that are hard to understand. I seek their scents and sounds, to enter deeply into their cupped, closed worlds because that is the struggle lying at the core of me. And I have learned that the only way to enter another's life is to find the vector points where my self and another self meet. If, one summer day a long time ago, I could have understood my heart as something petaled with blood or my bones as stems and roots, then perhaps the mandrake would have lived for me. Similarly, there is no way, I believe, to do the work of therapy, which is, when all is said and done, the work of relationship, without finding your self in the patient and the patient's self in you. In this way, rifts within and between might be sealed, and the languages of our separate lives might come to share syllables, sentences, whole themes that bind us together.

These, then, are not just stories of my patients; they are stories as well of myself, of interactions and conflicts, of the way one psychologist watches her past meet her present, coming to see herself in the complicated lattice of her patients' lives. These are stories of reflections and routes, including the route I have traveled to cope with my own psychiatric difficulties. Psychiatry and psychology, while paying homage to the significance of empathy and connection, have done little in the way of really revealing themselves and their practitioners, and connection is at least in part based on revelation, the stripping off of the mask. Especially in this time of managed care, more emphasis seems to be placed upon medication and the quick amelioration of symptoms, short-term work and privatized, profit-making clinics, than upon the lovely and mysterious alchemy that comprises the cords between people, the cords that soothe some terrors and help us heal.

In this book, I write about people I met at the very beginning of my career as a psychologist, when I was wobbly yet bold, as ambitious beginners often are. Perhaps some things I would think about or do differently now; perhaps not. One thing remains constant, though—my belief that neither pure insight nor pure behavioral change is solely transformative. I believe, rather, that therapy transforms when it is the slow learning about connection and separation, the visceral study of painful lacunae and blue links. I believe in a place, somewhere in the air, where my self and your self might meet, merging in what we might learn to call, at least for a moment, love.

ACKNOWLEDGMENTS

Thanks go to Ben Alexander, Molly Froelich, Liza Graver, Ed Harutunian, Joyce Mandell, William Oksner, Veronika Requat, Lisa Schiffman, Audrey Schulman, and Tracy Slater, for the friendship that softens the hard work of writing; also, to my writers' group, Mary Clark, Pagan Kennedy, and Karen Propp; to Susan Baur, whose work as a psychologist and a writer has so inspired and influenced me; to my agent, Kimberly Witherspoon, and her associate, Maria Massie; to Renana Meyers of Random House, and of course to Kate Medina, my Random House editor, whose support and encouragement have meant more to me than I can say.

CONTENTS

WELCOME
TO MY
COUNTRY

WELCOME TO
MY COUNTRY

Summer, ninety-five degrees, the street in East Boston where the residence for chronic schizophrenics is sits dead and silent in the heat. I am new at this, my doctoral training just finished. And I'm trying to think like a schizophrenic already, before I even have interviewed for the job at the Bates House; I'm attempting to enter what I believe will be a completely foreign place. Imagining psychosis, I see the leaves on the trees have gone brown and curled, the flowers are on fire; light glares and screeches in a shadowless world.

I ring the bell to the front door and a fat sweating boy, his face a mash of pimples, answers.

"I am here to see Dr. Siley," I say, glancing down at the newspaper clipping in my hand, where the job advertisement has sweated off in a Rorschach black. The pimply-faced boy stares and stares at me. I can tell, from his fatness and sweat, a patient. Then he reaches out and touches my neck. I flinch back from his hand. "What's wrong?" he hisses at me, spittle foaming in the corners of his lips. "You don't like me, you don't like me, you don't like me?" He sings more than says it, and I don't know what to say. I want to say, "I'm sorry." I want to say, "Don't you know it's not polite to touch someone before you know them?" I want to say, "You scare me." But instead I repeat, my voice tight, "I'm here to see Dr. Siley. Could you please get him for me?" The boy backs away. My very first contact with a patient has gone cold. "Dr. Siley," he wails, running down the cool hall of the institution. "Dr. Siley, some new shrink is here. Watch out for her. She's an alien. She has no bones in her neck."

So begins my work with the chronic schizophrenic population. I am an alien to them and they to me. I am hired by the director of the all-male residential unit to conduct group therapy for six of the patients once a week. During both my master's-level work in psychology at Harvard and my doctoral-level work at Boston University, I took courses on psychopathology. I've read not only the academic texts but the personal accounts as well, books like *I Never Promised You a Rose Garden* and *Autobiography of a*

Schizophrenic Girl. But none of this is enough to prepare me for the conundrums of working with these men. They appear to be the grotesques of this world, burdened by the most horrifying psychiatric illness known to humankind. As W. Hall, G. Andrews, and G. Goldstein have written, "Schizophrenia is to psychiatry what cancer is to medicine: a sentence as well as a diagnosis." Anyone who agrees to work with the chronic schizophrenic agrees to take on a supposedly hopeless case. This is what you are taught, what the research says. This is what my first group indicates.

My first group. Six men, all of whose charts I've read prior to actually meeting them. I watch as they file into the group room. They say their names one by one when I ask, and as they do I match up names and faces with the information I've gleaned from records.

There is Tran, nicknamed Moxi, a small, cocoa-colored Vietnamese who came to this country after the war, and who bows to invisible Buddhas all day in the corridors. There is Joseph, with a mangy beard, a green-and-khaki combat helmet he puts on the pillow next to him when he sleeps. Charles is forty-two years old and dying of AIDS. Lenny once stood naked in Harvard Yard and recited poetry. Robert believes fruits none of us can see are exploding all around him. And then there is Oscar, 366 pounds, and claiming constant blow jobs from such diverse females as the Queen of England and Chrissy, the Shih Tzu dog next door.

Oscar slogs into the group room, groans, lowers himself onto the floor, and lies there with his hairy belly bloating up.

"I am," I say, my voice cracking from fear (for I have never done this kind of work before; all my other patients have been violent or sad or scared but not . . . not . . . *this*), "your new group therapist. We'll be meeting once a week to talk things over, see how your lives are going, confront problems, think up solutions, play some games, even. How does that sound?"

Silence. Oscar, on the floor, appears to be asleep. Surprisingly delicate snores issue from his thick lips. The other men sit pressed against the walls or staring into their own squares of space as though they are strangers riding a train. And yet some of them have been living together in this institution for as long as seven years. As I get more acquainted with these people, I will come to understand how they almost always dwell in such silence. At mealtimes, or in the common room, they sit rocking, tracing imaginary figures in the air, lecturing on astrophysics to an invisible audience of esteemed colleagues, while in some place I cannot get to, comets explode and suns warp into white dwarves. The men's worlds are so far away from me and from one another that only occasionally will they reach out to filch a cigarette from someone next to them, moments later hunching back into themselves and collapsing into private giggles.

But I don't know any of this yet. I'm still brand new. I look around at my drooling patients. My mind charges over techniques, hovers, herds—how can I get them to interact? The silence thickens and I can hear, coming from outside, the dry gratings of insects in the summer heat.

Finally Joseph clears his throat, takes off his combat helmet, and stares deeply into its hollow. "What's in there, Joseph?" I ask. "What's in your helmet?"

"Blood be gone and hell swell sabooose," he says. "A girl curve feminine adventure."

I struggle to think of what to say. What part of this do I understand? What part can I, or any of the other group members, connect to? A girl curve? An adventure? I decide to let it go. "And, Charlie," I say, "can you tell me anything about yourself?"

"Char*les*," he cries. "No not Charlie but Char*les* Char*les* Char*les*." He bites into his lip and swings his head so violently I am reminded of a long time ago, when I went to the aquarium and saw a shark with a fish in the barbs of its teeth, the shark's flat silver head whipping back and forth as its prey's body burst. "Charles Charles Charles," he keeps repeating.

"Charles," Lenny, a black man, sings from the other side of the room. Lenny has skin the color of deep coal, his limbs long with rippled muscles rooted in them. Lenny looks so healthy, his body speaking the bones and sinews that stretch inside it. Surely, I think, this man will make some sense.

"Oh, Charles," Lenny says, looking not at Charles but resolutely up at the ceiling, "you need a protegé like Henry Collins. I have my protegé, Henry Collins, and if I don't go to Chelsea he stays with me and helps me not to be a pimp. I was once a pimp but before that my name is Cuppy."

"Cuppy?" I say to Lenny, squinting. "Your name is Cuppy?"

"Sometimes," Lenny says. "That depends on the fog."

It is useless, I think to myself during the first few weeks of the group, to try to get these men to connect with one another or myself, because connections between human beings depend at least partly on words, and the words of the schizophrenic are terribly skewed. The schizophrenic speaks a mumbo-jumbo language psychologists call a "word salad," nouns and verbs, fragments from the past, snippets of dreams all tossed into the lush wet mess. Sometimes beautiful sparks of sense do fly out, and other times bizarre but poetic hallucinations—the man with the blue ears who sleeps on the ceiling, miraculous cures that curl from test tubes foaming inside someone's head. You look for these swaths of sense and rhythm and, as you would any good wave, you try to ride it, but too often it fizzles into foam and you find yourself washed up in a tangle of mental kelp.

The staff in this unit, many of whom are highly experienced, having worked with the chronic schizophrenic population for many years, advise me to forget about doing "deep work"—work that either focuses on the patients' own internal worlds or attempts to foster real relationships among them—and I have no trouble agreeing. For one thing, my own training as a psychologist has stressed only behavior management with the schizophrenic, downplaying and even rejecting out of hand any other kind of psychotherapy. This may be because we know, from studies of schizophrenics' biochemical processes and brain structure, that such patients operate so far from the folds of the golden cortex, the most they can usually master are low-level self-care skills. Treatment for the chronic schizophrenic—and the academic training of the psychologist who will deliver such treatment—swerves away from explorations of hallucinations and delusions, or from the fostering of relational bonds, and focuses on what are called ADLs—Activities of Daily Living—how to budget your money, how to dress, how to take your medication on time, how to make a meal.

Each Friday, the six of us staff meet in the small front office. "Moxi isn't using soap when he showers," Bill, one of the counselors, says. "We need to address that issue with him."

"Oscar is eating too much pizza. Who here wants to help him count his calories?"

The meetings last only an hour but it feels more like four. Time drags on as we discuss getting Joseph to the dentist because his teeth are rotting—and fail to focus on the more interesting fact that he feels minnows swimming in his stomach—and as we talk about Robert and his med schedule, ignoring his fear of exploding fruits. Perhaps we do this because we don't understand fruits that splatter and stain a world none of us knows how to reach.

And perhaps we do this because every one of us who works at the inpatient unit is wedded to the belief that the schizophrenic, given his rotting neuronal pathways, the drought or deluge of dopamine in his brain, cannot think about higher-level concerns, like love and beauty, the swellings of intimate sex. It would be like trying to teach Dostoevski to a three-year-old, logarithms to an Alzheimer's sufferer.

But how did this belief come to be, I wonder? After all, a long time ago, in Freud's Vienna, the crazy man was seen as someone closer to creativity, van Gogh's stars stuffed in his twilit skull. Earlier in the century, Harold Searles wrote extensively on the emotional life of schizophrenics and the importance of therapy that honored and explored these feelings. I trace the loss of such views—the loss of the belief that schizophrenics are in need of complex emotional or relational-based interventions—to the rise in the 1950s of humanistic psychology and Abraham Maslow. Maslow, with his Hierarchy of Basic Needs, helped us to stop thinking so much about repression and to start thinking about actualization. According to Maslow, we all want to actualize ourselves, but only a few of us are able to do so. Before we can focus on higher-level needs—which include as core components emotional insight, love, and connections with others—we must be free first from hunger, thirst, and illness, and then from threats that endanger either psychological or physiological survival.

Maslow's model was linear, and it (along with behaviorism, trait psychology, and the increasing popularity of neuropsychology) may have contributed to the contemporary treatment philosophy of schizophrenics by suggesting that an ability to even consider issues like love and intimacy must be preceded by adequate shelter and a stable mind relatively free from interpersonal or intrapsychic threats. In Maslow's model, the very weight of a psychotic illness, with its attendant terrors and confusions, would probably subsume strivings of a higher sort.

And yet, as I begin to listen to the men in my group, as week after week goes by, I think I start to see glimmers of higher-level capabilities. Oscar's delusions have an awful lot to do with girlfriends who live on Pluto and land on rooftops when they wish to visit him. He tells me that in the night his seven hundred Chinese wives pay him visits, slipping in through the windows. And Joseph often babbles on and on about a mistress and two kids in Brighton who the staff tell me have never existed. Do these delusions, I wonder, possibly reflect a mature desire for intimacy in such seemingly immature minds? I'm not sure. I back up, wade forward, check, and test. What is it? How can I define it? In their tossed-up word salads I sometimes catch glimpses of continuous themes, diced-up apples of desire, green leaves of love. I want to go there, tread through those gardens.

It is late August now, and I've been leading the group for two months. Given the nature of my training, for two months I've been resisting a tread through the gardens. Instead I've been trying to dodge and weave through the spitballs of images these men throw at me, and I am tired. The heat has not yet broken over the city. Day after day it rises like a dream, caping the silver skyscrapers, trapping the smog so it drapes a drab brown over all our bridges. Sometimes when I step outside after work, the people hurrying to and fro on the sidewalk look like spirits to me, sad sweating ghosts from an underground world. Pieces of madness cling to me like lint and I can't shake them off. I am tired of the bizarreness of my patients, more tired still of trying to ignore their hallucinations and to focus, instead, on money and meds and keeping the shirt stain-free. When Lenny tells me in group he is communing with a woman who is also a paintbrush, I say to him, as I've been trained, "No, Lenny. There are no women who are also paintbrushes in this group. Why don't you tell all of us what you actually mean? Why don't you stop slumping, sit up, and button your shirt?" When Joseph tells the group he has shot seven soldiers in World War One, I say, "You have never been in World War One. You are here in this room. With all of us now. Tell us what your plans for the weekend are and why you have overslept three days in a row." Doing this work is like being the goalie in a soccer game; over and over again the swift kicks of craziness come at you, and over and over again you try to deflect them, or better yet, take the air right out of the ball.

And I am tired, and my own life has become a little boring, devoid of fantasy, flat. I think I need a new boyfriend, a dash of spice and sex. At night I drive to Bradlees because it stays open late, and I try on the wildest, craziest clothes I can—a jungle-patterned skirt and cowboy boots with red tassels, a little slip of a sundress that shows the dangerous dip between the breasts. In this way, I enter another place, something that may be closer to where my patients are, and at the same time rebelliousness kicks up in me. "Ha!" I think. "Activities of Daily Living. Give me a break."

And that may be why, when, a few days later, Oscar announces a spaceship has landed on his enormous belly, I break down. "All right," I say, looking around the room, eyeing the door and hoping it's closed so none of the other staff can hear, "why don't we go for a ride in it, then? Let's go."

"Let's go!" the irrepressible Lenny shouts, jumping up and down.

"Where?" I say, and indeed I mean it. I am thinking of the diced-up apples of desire, the green leaves of love. What about these things I hear in the schizophrenic's dream talk? Will the spaceship take us closer to such themes, the ones Maslow perches near the top of his hierarchy and that the schizophrenic is supposedly incapable of grasping?

Lenny strides across the room and eases down on the floor right next to Oscar. He takes his deep-black hand and lays it on top of Oscar's swollen white stomach. The hand sits there like a black star in a white sky, some sort of weird reversal.

"Move in," I say, looking around to the rest of my group members. "Charles," I say, "move in, right up next to Oscar. You too, Moxi," I say to the little man who, week after week, sits hunched and rocking in a corner, who won't move, won't speak, ever. Moxi is the most closed-off of all. He is missing three fingers and one testicle because the voice of Mother Mary told him to cut them off. The most he will do in group is mumble a yes or a no. "You too, Moxi," I say a little louder.

The men all eye me, something alert in their usually slack faces; they edge forward on their seats. I edge out of my own seat and sit on the floor, so close I can see the rise and fall of Oscar's belly, on his face the bubbles of sweat that seep from large red pores.

"A spaceship," I repeat to Oscar. "On your belly right now. To take us into your world." The rest of the men creep forward, sit Indian-style in a circle around him. It's the closest I've ever seen any of them get to one another. "We are going into the spaceship,"

I say, "and we're all riding up. What do we see, Oscar? Where are we?"

Lenny still has his hand on Oscar's belly, and now he is moving it back and forth, rubbing. Oscar, his voice flat and thick, begins to speak.

"Sheba," he says. "We are going to see Sheba. She lives up there, my girl does, in the sky. She is a star. She eats leg of lamb without the skin. And octopus."

"Octopus," Joseph says. "Freaky."

"Sheba is your girl," I say.

"I have hundreds of girls," Oscar replies, "all over the sky. Definitively they are albinos. They keep me company. They love me."

"They love you," I say and, thinking of the overweight unloved-by-girls Oscar, something sad rises up in me. I feel my own voice grow low, whispery. The room seems darker, even though the summer sun burns like an ember in the white sky outside. Shadows, sexy shadows, ripple and sway on the walls.

"They love him," Joseph says, and there is something keening in his voice. "I myself am waiting for my wife in Brighton. She keeps me good company. Sometimes she sits on my head."

"And the albino," Oscar says. His eyes are closed and our spaceship swims and spins. "She has quite a cunt."

"It is hard," Lenny announces, "to get into a cunt. Especially if it's not broken in. But once you're in, you fall out so fast. My protegé, Henry Collins, agrees."

"Falling out falling out," Charles murmurs. He rocks back and forth and his silver hair glows like some sort of outer-space strobe. And we rise and spin and at the same time I think we are closer to the ground than we've ever been.

"Landing," Lenny says, and he takes his hand and slaps the floor—*splat*. We all jump, startled. The dream is broken. The albinos shimmer away.

One by one the men shuffle back to their usual seats, each distanced from the others again. They start their rocking and tapping, separated in their own spheres. But for just a moment they did join together, and I went with them.

So perhaps there *is* a bridge from their private worlds into one another's, and into mine. Made of delicate wrought iron that bridge is, studded with winged gargoyles, something strange but strong enough to survive the winds of insanity. The men look so lonely to me, each one sitting far apart and mute again, staring into his own square of air. But when we sat on the floor and spoke of women, the longings for company and kin, I could connect to that. We could, each one of us, connect to that. Crazy or sane, we all know the desire for skin touching skin, or brain rubbing brain as minds meet.

Out on the street, businessmen, teenagers, girls in sundresses—the whole city parades past. The patients turn to watch with something aching in their eyes. Most of them have lived in the isolation of institutions for years. I think of Charles, who has never worked but is saving every penny from his government check for a briefcase, some small sliver of the culture he can clutch. And as we watch from our side of the screen, a lady with a rose tattoo on her shoulder prances past. "Hello hello," Joseph croons, tapping on the glass, "hello hello," and then his speech turns into salad. "Oh golden boats and pods." He pauses, eyes rolled back, fighting for the words he means. He tries again. "Heaven of flying dirt," he shouts, turning once more to look at the lady, who has disappeared around the city block. "Harsh under the wall," he splutters. He grips his fist and shakes his head, trapped in his wordbound illness.

On the floor, Oscar groans. He taps three times on his belly. "We suffer," he says. "We suffer to speak so."

I want to help them get back into that spaceship. The more I think about it, the clearer it becomes to me, these men's pivotal concerns with connection, how to get it, how to hold it, how to mourn its loss. Although their desires are oftentimes expressed in lusty ways, I don't believe they are motivated by something as simple as lust. The longing for the briefcase, the sensitivity to language and frustration over its loss, the simple touches and aches in their faces—these things lead me to believe their stretches for connections are occurring at more complex levels, are rooted in the need to belong, to participate in the wider world. At the same time, though, I can't help but wonder if I'm not imposing those concerns on them, trying to grid my more advanced meaning system onto the mush of their minds. I go to the library one evening after work and look up the literature on delusions. There are articles on delusions of grandeur and paranoia, but nowhere does the literature mention delusions that weave around the themes of longing and loss, of great space and tundra. Why? I wonder. Is it that the schizophrenic experience seems so bizarre to us, we can't imagine such a patient might be suffering from something as common as loneliness? As highbrow as existential anomie? I don't think I would be so simplistic as to say that schizophrenia is *caused* by existential anomie or a baser brand of loneliness, but its consequence seems to be a heightened sense of isolation and a keen desire to connect, finding fusion through fantasy, the only way the illness allows.

This is just a hypothesis, but I decide to go with it. I decide, for the time being, to abandon the ADL stuff in group, the *buttonyourshirtsitupstraightwhywon't-youtakeyourmedsremembertopickupthebathmat,* and assume they are capable of more. I try to build a group that is explicitly a social sphere. I wonder whether or not, given guidance, these men will be able to learn how to form connections to one another that break through the membrane of their own madness. And if they can form connections, enter into relationships, as they seemingly desire—the desire their delusional systems speak of—I wonder what kinds of relationships they will actually have.

I make the group more activities-oriented because I believe relationships are best formed through the sharing of common contexts. And I make the group kinesthetic because I suspect only physical movement will be powerful enough to propel my patients out of their separate spheres. Sometimes it works and sometimes it doesn't. We have a remarkably successful pizza party one afternoon, the men managing, after an hour of in-depth negotiation, to order sausage and pepperoni toppings and walk down to the pizza parlor and pick up the pies, and then scarfing down the fruits of their labor while sitting around the kitchen table in what resembled a family meal.

I have to shed some of my own inhibitions and shake myself up. I have been trained, after all, to sit in an office and communicate with my clients through streamlined sentences. Now I must learn to sing.

" 'Leaving on a Jet Plane'?" I suggest, remembering that tune from my childhood.

" 'Summer Wind,' " Oscar says, and to my surprise he sits up, does a wonderful rendition of Sinatra, a song full of golden sands and blue skies. The men blink, open their eyes. Robert strides across the room and offers Oscar his fist for a microphone; the song slides down into Robert's hand, and when it is finished, Robert presses his fingers to his face, stays that way for the rest of the time.

The group, like a waking baby animal, blinks, stretches, and mewls. There is nothing especially dramatic about this, just subtle snatches of seconds when hands are pressed to cheeks, when songs come from a mouth open one moment and then snapped closed the next. And, to be sure, there are long periods when nothing seems to work, when the men will not talk or interact at all. There is, yes, still much rocking, tapping, dreaming, drooling. But just a little something seems to shift. A song here or there. And I am a bit proud when the counselor Sophie stops me in the hall on my way out of work one day and says, "Things seem lighter around here. The other day Lenny barged into the office and serenaded staff with 'Mack the Knife.' "

I bring in pastels and large sheets of fresh white paper, ask the men to draw a gift they would most like to give another member of the group. Some of the men roll the pastels against their faces, eyes half closed. Lenny picks a deep red color, sweeps it across the page, and then leans back to peer at the crimson line of life. "Ahhh," he says to himself. "Ahhh, yessss. Yesssss." He uses the crayon to draw an elaborate design in the air and then goes over to Charles, slowly traces a thick vein in Charles's neck. Charles, like a silver cat, arches his neck to the touch.

With the windows open, the sheets of paper flutter and smartly smack in the end-of-summer breeze. The men seem invigorated, except for Moxi, who still sits hunched and rocking in his private corner. Robert draws what he tells me is a whorehouse, prances across the room, and plops the paper into Joseph's lap. Joseph salutes him and says a crisp commander "thank you." Lenny draws what he calls a ravioli and sends it to Oscar. Oscar, in his usual repose on the floor, manages to turn on his side, stretch out an arm, and draw a picture of his mother. "Who do you want to give it to?" I ask.

He doesn't answer. Instead he looks down at the few crude lines he has drawn. He says, "I am afraid. Afraid of when she dies. Who will take care of me? No one else is left in my family. It's why I have Sheba and the girls in my head. The crazy thoughts and the girls are better than nothing."

Moments like these make my work rewarding. Moments when the clouds of confusion clear away and the seemingly incapable patient choruses through with a gem of sense. Into my memory at moments like these comes the comet I saw when I was a little, little girl. It was late at night, and I was in a garden in the Caribbean, surrounded by strange blooms I had never seen before, mysterious pursed and drooping plants with tongues and shining white stars in their centers. And a hand (whose hand? A dream hand with shadow fingers) tilted up my chin and a voice (whose voice? My father's voice) told me to look into the sky, for there was a flower stranger even than the ones on this earth—a comet flaring from the darkness, its tail a flutter of fiery petals. And the voice, my father's voice, told me the comet had come tonight and would not do so again for a long time. And watching Oscar on the floor cross the wrought-iron bridge with the gargoyles on it is the same as seeing that comet, a bright burst, something sad and wonderful, loss poised inside the single sparks of his words. I smile.

"I am lonely," Oscar says, still clear. He plucks a brown pastel out of the box and speed-sketches an empty skull. "It's what my head looks like without Sheba and the albino girls," he says. Suddenly he looks straight up at me, winks. "Girl," he says, "wanna go under the sprinkler with me?"

Outside on the lawn a sprinkler is fanning back and forth, spattering water onto the parched grass. "Can't," I say. "But if you're lonely, why don't you ask one of the men in this group for a hug?"

"What are we, homos?" Charles snarls. He is so thin from the AIDS that the veins in his neck flash as he speaks, and Lenny's crimson cord jumps. I wonder if Charles is homosexual but can't admit it.

"Go on," I say to Oscar. "No *real* man turns down a dare."

Oscar looks around. "Hey," he says, hefting himself up so he is close to Robert. "Hey, wacko. Wanna give your buddy a hug?"

Brave men, yes, learning to touch, learning to love in these treacherous times of theirs.

In November, Charles begins to die. He is timely. He loses his strength just as the last of the leaves wisp down from the trees and the bare barbs of branches jut into the air. When I wake up in the morning and see the silver rime of frost on the grass, I think of Charles shining in his illness. He grows so very thin the tracery of bones becomes visible and his eyes sink into crepuscular hollows. Sores splutter open on his skin, weep a watery red liquid he won't wash away. Staff put on latex gloves to clean him.

One day when I am up on the second floor of the ward gathering the men from their rooms because it's group time, I walk in on Charles naked. I see loveliness mixed with horror, the spine standing out like a string of pearls just beneath the thinnest sheath of skin, and then blossoms of sores on his arms and buttocks, all wet and fresh. "We can't keep him here," Sophie says in staff meeting. "We're endangering all the other patients."

Bill, another staff member, finds Charles crumpled on the stairs a few days later, and an ambulance comes to take him away. The men won't watch. They scatter into the dayroom or their own bedrooms, stubbornly stare into the air and trace invisible figures. "Say good-bye to Charles," Bill says as the stretcher is wheeled out.

"Who'll take care of him?" Oscar asks, and then, as though thinking of his own mother, he turns away and starts to rock and tap. Too painful, this is.

Too painful, this is, because Oscar's question is so apt. Charles is taken to the hospital, but when nothing can be done for him there, he is removed to an inner-city hospice to die. He has no family, no friends. No mother or brother or aunt steps forward to pay for extra medical care or plan a burial. Sophie burns a candle for Charles in the office. The entire ward takes up a collection and we put in what we can. The patients understand this radical aloneness. They drop in their dimes.

A few days after Charles has been removed to the hospice, Sophie finds Robert standing in the entrance to Charles's old room, screaming. Then the sound stops. All sounds stop and an eerie silence settles over the ward. When I bring in pastels, the men won't touch them. When I suggest pizza, they grunt and rock and talk about Sheba. Over and over again Oscar sucks on his fist in a frenzy. I can't reach the men anymore, nor they me. "Wind, wind in my head," Robert moans, "the world disappearing, eaten up by photons. My hand is swelling and she hit me. Hit me!"

He looks up at me and I can't help but wonder if he is asking me to hit him, some sharp swat that would bolt him back into the world. This, I think, must be the most horrifying part of mental illness, the few glimpses you get of connection, and then the psychosis taking over with such a fierceness that lights go down and the world as we know it shatters like a fragile glass globe. I don't want to think of such terrors. And I'm scared to stand so close to the raw grief of these lives.

All I can really do is watch helplessly as the men drool and slip from their lives, from one another, back into their separate spheres. I don't know how much Charles's fading has to do with the group's fading. I don't know how close the men were even able to feel to Charles himself. But what I do know is that two things are dying here, one man and one community, whose connections are crumbling as they barely began to coalesce.

And I do know now that the schizophrenic, in his better moments, is capable of some sorts of connections. These patients, I have learned through my work in the group, feel deep erotic connections to their own imaginary brides. And, when treatment encourages it, they can also feel and act upon the chummy, friendly sorts of unions that include the complex recognition of self and other, and that, therefore, make the world a warmer place.

But not during these days of dying. The heat has broken, that's for sure. Outside the air feels cold on my skin, smacks with the smell of snow. I go to the supermarket after work these days; it, too, stays open late. Many things hurt. The fruits are blooming in

their bins, but it's an ugly sight, those scarlet tomatoes and bruised purple eggplants swollen in frozen
sleeps. Good-bye.

"Good-bye" is what we call our poem when we
write it in the group. The men say the statements; I
write them down and give some organization. I ask
each man to contribute a few lines. For some
moments they step back out of their insanity and
oblige me. They say about Charles:

> He used to eat piles of sardines
> He slept a lot
> I miss him at the table when we had pizza
> He kept to himself but
> He was a key in the hole of this house
> I had a lot of personal dependence on him
> I miss the very first thing he said to me:
> He said, "You clean steps well."
>
> I will remember how I called him Okar and he
> Called me Doink. He'd go, "Hey, Doink!"
> And he moved slowly
> I miss him because I am losing a friend
> I'm thinking about him with no one
> No one
> Does he have any relationships? Any family?
> Or were we, here,
> Everything?

And that is all. No more words. No more songs or
giving of gifts. Snow starts, falling from the dry sky

like shavings of bone. Often I find myself thinking of Charles lying in the hospice bed, his yellowing skull and sparse hair. And then I think about who he once was, that silver shark, flat head swinging, body of supple muscle.

One day, a week before Charles finally dies, I bring a rubber ball into group. "OK," I say. "Everyone up. Stand in a circle."

"Not unless Robert comes," Lenny mumbles.

"Robert can come," I say, looking over toward Robert, who has his hands jammed over his ears. "Take your hands away from your ears, Robert," I shout, "and join our circle."

We make a circle, even Moxi.

"Whoever has the ball," I explain, "cannot toss it to someone else unless he asks a question of that person first. And whoever receives the ball has to answer the question and cannot throw the ball without asking a new question. In this way, we will reestablish our friendships and continue to get to know one another better."

The men stare at me, flat-eyed. I throw the ball to Joseph. "Joseph," I say, "what are you most afraid of?"

Joseph catches the ball. "Chips," he says. "Chips the CIA have planted in my brain." He throws the ball to Oscar. "Oscar," he says, "are you—?" but then he splutters into panicked giggles and can't finish the question. Oscar doesn't even bother catching the ball. It bounces off his blubbery chest and dribbles into the center of the circle.

"OK!" I say, all fake enthusiasm. "Let's start again!" I trot into the center of the circle, pick the ball back up. But I feel ridiculous.

I bounce the ball, thinking. "Robert," I say, tossing it again. "Who do you most love?" Robert catches the ball, cradles it, and won't let go. "Throw the ball, Robert," I say. "Go on." He throws the ball then, but backward, over his head, so it swerves outside the circle, and we're all left looking at one another, looking at nothing.

I sigh. "It's hard for everyone," I say at last. "Maybe you are all too upset about Charles."

"Nuh-uh," says Oscar. He slinks back into his customary slump on the floor. "We're not upset about Charles. We're all like Charles. None of us can die, because we're already dead."

And then each member of the circle, as though on cue, slumps to the floor. Only Moxi is left standing.

Moxi's eyes tick around the room, tick back and forth over the fallen bodies. His little broom of a mustache quivers. "No," he says. It is maybe the first word he has ever said in group. "No!" he says again. "Not true! Not true!" His English is laden with a heavy Vietnamese accent. "No no no," he chants. "I come here all the way from Vietnam. I have family. Family!"

"Who's in your family?" I ask, thinking of the chart I read on Moxi, in which it was reported his father and three sisters were bombed to death in his village during the war.

"Here!" he says, his eyes still swinging around the room, lighting on me and then on the other slumped men. "Here, here. In America! My family is in this place, this room. Now!" he shouts. "Here!"

And then Moxi bursts forth. He splits his separate sphere. I don't know why Moxi once put a knife to his penis but perhaps it had to do as much with the imagined voice of Mother Mary as with the need to cut away the thick skin of madness and maleness that prevents unions from happening with any ease.

And Moxi bursts forth. He unzips his fly, and with his hips shrugs off his pants. The pants fall to the floor, showing us, beneath, the single wrinkled testicle hanging like a chestnut on a winter tree. Moxi cups his penis in his hand.

"Oh, man," Lenny says, rolling around on the floor. "That is definitely not a cunt."

"No," I say, my own head spinning with shock (disrobing in the middle of group? What do I make of this? Should I stop it? How?). "No," I repeat, and suddenly something is singing in my voice. All the men are looking up now, sitting up now, shaking off the snow of a long sleep. I can practically see the white powder falling from their shoulders. "No, it's not a cunt," I say. "It's Moxi."

"I have many wounds," Moxi says. "I do them to myself when the buses go up the street the wrong way or the holy light speaks. I do them," he says, and pauses, sadness in his voice, "I do them to myself because I must."

Then Moxi walks up to Oscar and points to a raised welt on his thigh. Shaped like a crescent, a pale puffed pink. "Touch it," Moxi orders, but before Oscar can, he whips around to face Robert. "Touch it," he says again.

Robert reaches up to touch it. His finger lingers on the crescent. Moxi's penis shivers and swells. "Yes," Moxi says, backing away. "Yes."

"Touch it," he says, toddling up to Lenny, pointing to what looks like a self-inflicted burn on his knee. Lenny lifts a long elegant black finger and then, like a pianist pressing a key, lands lightly on the wound. I swear a sound springs out.

A heavy hush fills the room now. Outside the winter sky is darkening and a thin blade of moon slices up into the sky. As we touch Moxi's wounds, the group comes alive again, resurrects itself, the red gashes, the fire in the flesh. And somewhere, on the other side of this city, Charles with the blossoms on his body is rising too, and when I look out the group-room window I see a shadow there, a shark swimming up the street toward me, his body a thrusting curve, and then a sad man with silver hair tapping on the glass. Tap tap. *Let me in. Let me in.* The dead are starting to speak.

And the little man, half-naked, begins to dance. The rest of the men come together, draw in. They hum and clap in time to a rhythm and we are all a part of it, some sacred strip dance of death and life and the links between bodies—my fingers, your toes, my cut, your crying. Moxi sways. He rolls up his shirt sleeve and, crooning, points to more charred spots on his skin. "Here," he says. "And here too." He points with precision, insists that we see his hurts, insists, yes, that we see *him,* and some love gets built around his bared body.

Still naked, Moxi kneels and begins to draw a female figure.

"Who is she?" Robert whispers.

"She is a lady," Moxi answers. "A lady from Vietnam who I want to marry but who is already married."

He looks like he is going to cry now as he scurries about the room rolling down his shirt sleeves, pulling back on his pants. Then he does cry, standing in the center of the group room. He puts his hand over his heart and starts to sing in Vietnamese. His voice and the ballad have a mournful, ancient feel, each word with some weeping inside.

"Moxi, that was beautiful," I say. "What does the song mean?"

"I love a lady who doesn't love me; I am lost, oh, so lost," Moxi says. "That's what the song means." And then he sings it again, louder, his voice lovely and quavering.

"You are so lonely, aren't you, Moxi," I say.

"Yes, and I am so sad because Oscar won't shake my hand."

Oscar, leaning back against the wall, hands folded on the bubble of his belly, opens one eye as slowly as a lizard in the sun. "Huh?" he says.

"You won't shake my hand," Moxi repeats, agitated now.

"Don't always feel like it, Moxi," Oscar says. "Sometimes I'm just too tired."

"But you want Oscar to shake your hand, Moxi," I say.

"Everyone to shake my hand," Moxi says.

"Can we shake Moxi's hand?" I ask the group.

"Yeah," says Lenny. "And then we go to a whorehouse."

"OK," I say to Moxi. "Go on. We want to shake your hand."

Moxi skips around the room, nimble, hopeful. He cavorts and bows. He shakes each man's hand with pride. "Welcome to my country," he says to each person as he clasps him in a handshake. "Welcome to my country."

"Welcome," each one of us says back.

What country does he mean? I wonder. For sure there is something a little crazy about all of this, but also so appropriate. I think of the empty skull Oscar once drew and how we are, in this group, trying to learn to go through bone and enter those private sockets where our separate brains sit. And I think, Dr. Maslow, no matter how sick we are, how strained we are, we never stop wanting such closeness. We never lose the language altogether. Sheba is in the sky. She stretches out her red robes and takes a sad boy in. Charles, right this minute, is wandering in a land we will try and try to reach. A spaceship swims out of his dark and Moxi leads us in. We go up and up, past Sirius and Jupiter, past a dancing dog and a child's old playpen, a stained bib and a striped beach ball, until at last we land on a planet where Robert's fruits grow on all the trees, where comets flare above plants in mysterious gardens, plants that open their scary and lovely leaves. Here, in this group, the men pick the plants from a foreign world. They pile sparks and blooms in their baskets, and later, when they get back down to Earth, they will try to give them out as gifts to you and you and me. Welcome to my country.

STRIPTEASE

A personality disorder is one of the more troubling diagnoses a mental-health worker can give to someone seeking relief from suffering. Unlike a neurosis, viewed as a set of curable symptoms, or a psychosis, increasingly believed to be the result of a trigger-happy brain in need of mere medication, the personality-disordered individual is seen as close to hopeless, beyond the reach of either drugs or healing dialogue. The man or woman with such a diagnosis is thought of as a kind of blighted being, the udder of a cow on the belly of a gazelle, flippers on the side of a skunk. What can you do with this mishmash except try to soothe its confused cries?

I'd been working on a residential unit for chronic schizophrenics for a few months now, and had decided to add fifteen hours a week in the outpatient clinic located at the back of the building, overlooking a small oval of green surrounded by an intricate wrought-iron fence. Peter came through that fence and into the clinic's front doors in late autumn. He was diagnosed by the intake worker as having an antisocial personality disorder—in short a sociopath, a deviant—and I was now assigned to work with him for an undefined length of time. When I first met him, he looked almost ridiculously tough, sitting in a sleeveless leather vest in the clinic's lobby, hair scrunched back in a ponytail, a cigarette dangling from his mouth. Tattoos coiled over his arms, bloomed on his bare chest.

Immediately I felt awkward in his presence. Perhaps I was experiencing some throwback to my high school days, when I longed to be liked by the cool and vicious popular kids, who stared at the world slant-eyed and wagged their Winstons in the teachers' faces. Around such a crowd I have always felt stout and dumpy, the dust from my ancestors' Jewish shtetl still settled on my skin. The day I met Peter I was wearing my usual working garb, a smocked dress, a pair of flats, my legs stubbly from hair I'd only half-shaved and perhaps a swatch of slip showing from beneath my hem.

As a therapist, I think I should be beyond these silly social embarrassments. I think I should at least be sufficiently beyond my own bodily insecurities to throw my full attention into the client's waiting lap, but I am not. Around Peter I was not, and the sense of shame he evokes in me, to this day, is part of our treatment story together.

My office at the time was windowless and so small we had to sit with our knees near brushing. I got ready to ask my usual orienting questions. Especially with a client like Peter, who makes rise in me my own archaic discomforts, these questions are like life rafts I throw myself, bright verbal floats I can cling to.

"Age?" I asked.

Instead of answering me, Peter gave a dramatic sigh. "Whew!" he said. "Have I been waiting for this day. I've seen six of you guys and so far no one's worked out. I need a doc who can really push me. I need to be challenged."

In my mind then I pictured a boxing ring, a hefty human in each corner, leather mitts poised for the punch.

"Challenged?" I asked. "Like how?"

"I've got my problems," Peter said, "and I can admit to them. The other six I went to just sat there and stared at me. I want someone who will give me feedback, make me see things in a whole new way."

"So what are these problems?"

Peter sat back, ran one hand over a large Indian-princess tattoo on his bicep. "Masturbation," he said gravely. "I can't stop."

"Can't—"

"Nope! Seven, eight, nine times a day. I have a very strong drive." He shook his head in wonder. He looked proud, like a little boy opening a toy chest to show me his magnificent seven-sail ship. Now he pulled a list out of his pocket and began to read. "Masturbation, pornography, aggression, defensiveness, pride, control. These are my character defects. Take porn: I love it, but the truth is I'd rather do it with a videotape than with my girlfriend, Joanne. We have huge beefs, huge," Peter said. "My anger is just"—he paused—"like I think I could kill her. I've killed a few people before, so I wouldn't put it past me." Peter was staring straight at me when he said this, testing my reaction.

"So why do you think you prefer porn to people?" I said, keeping my voice even despite the fact that I suddenly felt like fleeing.

"Don't get me wrong," Peter said. "I like Joanne. She's a real smoker. But I'll be honest—a picture's just a lot easier. No one you gotta talk to. No one to perform for or try to please. Just a completely quiet and beautiful bod . . ."

I thought of my own "bod" then and felt my breasts beneath my dress burn with shame.

For the rest of that session I gathered background information. Peter was thirty-two years old, had lived seven of those years on the street, drugging, knife-fighting, and stealing. During those years he slept beneath fire escapes and went in and out of prisons, where the beds were warmer, the dope cheaper. He had been clean now for half a decade, a really remarkable achievement that he attributed to his spirituality, a weird blend of mysticism and heavy metal. In his East Boston apartment, where he lived with Joanne, he had two special cupboards side by side. In one of them he kept his incense, tarot cards, and his books on palm reading; in the other he stored his collection of sadomasochistic videos and magazines. Oddly, this second cupboard was lined with floral contact paper left by a previous tenant.

They brought him satisfaction, these videos. A lot went on for him each day. Joanne was, as he said, a beautiful woman, but she was also unpredictable and self-absorbed, a series of seismic cycles he could not control. "Modern woman," he said, shaking his head. He told me he was from the old school, expected his girl to cook and clean, to have his fish on the table by six each night, expected dustless halls and sex where her moans were synchronized to his orgasms. When Joanne let him down in any of these areas, he got mad, really red-faced furious, so that he hauled her up against the wall, walloped her across the face; he felt so much sheer and irrational hate that he had to retreat to his room to watch his videos; they soothed him, these images of female flesh cut into, female flesh controlled, the man pumping with pride above her.

Just by writing these words I can feel Peter's anger, his gut lust to control. It is real to me, this hatred of the female form. In our first several sessions I tried to find the origins of this hate. For instance, Peter's father, a stonemason, dead now ten years. He went to work at six in the morning, returned home after eight each night, his face similar to the substances he worked with, features descending like ledges to a jutting chin nicked with a dimple. He would have been a handsome man, except his expression was so stern and his breath smelled; when his father was drunk, Peter imagined his father's breath took on the color of the liquor he swallowed, so he exhaled yellow on whiskey nights, neon green on Midori.

His father beat him, but the beatings were not as bad as the humiliation that went along with them. He remembers the strap, the hands that were like hatchets; however, the intensity of his tale lies for me in this image: a small boy pressed against a refrigerator white as a nuptial bedsheet, the man pressing against him, shouting at him; Peter could feel his father's groin, hot and hard, right in the nook between his thighs. He started to think of himself as having a nook there, a gross, gaping place. One day, when he was outside playing, he had a terrible fantasy. Peter was twelve years old now; he imagined his body was a girl's. In his mind he lifted dark mounds of dirt from the garden and molded them onto his flat chest, making breasts. Then he went further, cut into his own body; he saw himself pluck off his penis, peel his mouth from his face, and carefully place it between his legs, tweaking the tongue so the red tip lapped over the lips. He could feel his father close by him, possibly right behind him, watching this and getting aroused. Peter was disgusted, horrified. A sheen of sweat broke out on his forehead. Soon afterward he learned to fight, started to lift weights, running from the softness that is the requisite for all rapes.

I had, at first, a hard time dealing with Peter because he offended me. I understood his pornography obsession as a deflection of his own anxieties. So he wouldn't have to feel his fear, his memories of helplessness, he tried to control women. He wanted to whittle my sex, and therefore me, down to a tiny teacup he could lift to his suddenly powerful lips and sip. Now, understand, I am a woman who has spent much time aiming to please men. I am a woman who, in her adolescent days, denied herself food or threw it all up so she could fit into the airless image a man in her office was both struggling to possess and to shed at the same time. I remember the smell of myself as a starving girl, a frail, dry odor, like scorched grass, my limbs coated with hair. Because of these memories, it was impossible for me to like Peter, but I did feel deeply for him. After all, hadn't I once striven for his same goals, to control the random, fleshy facets of female life, to eradicate the weak part of the self who hurts and bleeds and feeds? In a sense we were both murderers and we were both crying out from our crimes.

During the first few weeks of our therapy together I began to feel the old shame about my body returning more strongly than it had in a while. Although Peter said he wanted help overcoming his pornography obsession (he was sometimes driven to watch five, six films a night) and to learn to understand and defuse his rages, he used his sessions to vent about Joanne's latest transgressions, and from there he would segue into paeans about "the perfect pussy," its size and smell. After a day when I'd seen Peter, I would go home and feel my flesh more heavily than ever. I often wanted to weep. And it was during this time that I noticed small black hairs growing up around my nipples. On the one hand, I wanted to pluck them out. On the other hand, I wanted to let them grow, lush like the marsh weeds that spring up in swamps.

My prescription was for Peter to learn, somehow, that being soft does not mean being molested or murdered, necessarily. And that softness is not only a requisite for rape but also the texture of soil and sheets and the tender, almost melting skin that covers the penis. To that end, I thought he should explore his wounds and weaknesses and thereby gain the knowledge that feeling them now, in a safe place, would not bring the humiliation he feared but the enriched humanity he claimed he wanted. He would have none of it, of course. While he came to therapy stating he ached for change, he remained, in his actions, dedicated to defensiveness. He all but brought rifles to our sessions. He ranted, swore, swung the verbal muzzle left, now right; his neck was almost beautiful, strung with gut, a trigger moving in his throat.

When we had been going at it for about two months, he told me a story that just about bowled me over.

The woods behind his childhood home divided his family's house from that of Teddy Swayez, a classmate. Peter was nine years old, and that day Teddy had promised him the use of his new red Tonka toy truck if only Peter would come over and play.

But when Peter got there, Teddy went back on his part of the bargain. The truck, nope, was not to be shared. Peter had walked all this way, had stumbled over tree roots, had opened himself to hope, only to find he was fooled.

He felt a curious, sick stirring in his stomach and between his legs as he watched that Swayez kid totally ignore him, moving the truck up and down a dirt pile, treaded tires leaving small slashes and scars in the sand.

So Peter went home, took his father's knife and some rope from the cellar, and made a gallows in the woods, using branches as a platform. "Boy have I got the coolest thing to show you," Peter said to Teddy. "You gotta come."

And then, when they were there, Peter said, "Look up." It was floating against the sky, the noose, very bright in the sunlight.

"Climb," Peter said, using his father's knife to persuade. He remembers this moment as being very fine, clearly etched, shadows cool as corpses on the ground, a cocoon in the niche of a tree, the glaze of snot on Teddy's blubbering lip. He used the blade on the kid's soft skin and had a sudden, jarring image of his mother, in the kitchen in the morning, wearing an apron and slicing through a warm bar of butter.

Teddy was up there; Peter positioned his head in place, kicked away the sticks, so all of a sudden Teddy swung, neck bunched in the noose . . .

I was leaning forward in my seat. I thought I might throw up. "Oh, Jesus," I said. "What happened?"

Peter snorted, sucked back some mucus into his throat. "The rope broke," he said. "I knew it would. It was already ragged as hell. I just wanted to scare him because I wouldn't be had. I *can't* be had; you see what I mean?"

I didn't say anything.

"You see what I mean?" he shouted, nodding his head in agitation.

"Yes, yes, I see what you mean," I said quickly. "It's horrible for you to have to endure any kind of humiliation or helplessness. The only way you know how to deal with it is by getting the person back even worse."

"That's the only way I know," Peter agreed. "Otherwise I feel like I'm just a doormat." He took an angry drag on his cigarette and then crushed it out in the ashtray, which was littered with the smushed remains of all Peter's butts.

"But do you think everyone in the world wants to treat you as a doormat? Was Teddy Swayez really trying to humiliate you, or was he just possibly feeling selfish at the moment you arrived? I mean, is every-one in the whole world just waiting for their chance to take advantage of Peter, abuse Peter in some way?"

"Absolutely," Peter said. "I know it."

"God. It must be tiring having to think that. You can never really let down your guard. Have you ever cried in front of someone, shown that you're scared, upset?"

Peter didn't say anything. For a moment I thought he looked sad. I had the urge to reach over, take him by his uptight shoulders, and shake him until I felt his muscles turn sap-soft and sweet, feel the rusty joints and junctures of his body loosen and liquid slip through.

A long silence settled between us; we were a cut cord, a swarm of static.

"Peter," I said, trying again, "as a kid, feeling any-thing but vengeful violence was dangerous, because your dad really did abuse you. But do you have to turn the whole world into him now? What would happen if, at this very moment, right here, you let me know what you were feeling? Try."

Silence.

"What's going on, Peter? My hunch is you won't be diminished by showing yourself, but you'll actually be a lot 'bigger' by allowing yourself to feel more."

"Oh, really?" Peter said. His tone sounded subtly sarcastic and curious at the same time.

"Why is it unsafe to feel anything but defensiveness or violence in this office? Do you think I'm going to take advantage of you?"

He smiled. Immediately I realized I'd made a blunder by allowing him the opportunity to sexualize our interaction.

"*You*, take advantage of me? Isn't it supposed to be the other way around?" He leaned back in his chair, lit another cigarette. I saw the smoke slide from his mouth, felt it wrap around me in a blue and gauzy cloud, decking me in the moving material of a see-through dress.

Mistrust is the fuel for so much mental pain, so many mental disorders. I am not talking here about the suspicions we sometimes have of one another, the distant but lurking sense that perhaps our lover lies to us, our best friend whispers behind our back. I am talking about a belief that betrayal inundates the atoms of the universe, is so woven into the workings of the world that every step is treacherous, and that below the rich mud lies a mine.

Peter believed that the bodies outside of him were missiles poised and poisonous. His aggressive, slit-

eyed stance is, without doubt, a typically male phenomenon. My eating disorder, the obsessive desire to
be thin thin thin and perfectly poisonously poised, is
a typically female phenomenon. But their shared
themes must not go unnoticed if the sexes are ever to
learn real compassion for each other. Peter and I were
both victims of our culture's fear of the feminine,
unable to lay down our system of weapons and
spread our legs open to life because we learned that in
this posture we would be shamed, not invigorated.
We did not know how to trust what we could not
dominate. In treating Peter, I came to remember with
eerie clarity the years and years of my own hostile
dieting—I am forcing myself to run ten miles under a
broiling summer sun; I am climbing the sixty stories
of my father's apartment building, footsteps slapping
echoes in the clammy concrete stairwell. I believed my
body was my enemy, every cell, unless vigilantly
starved by exercise, eager to add layer upon layer of
crude fat.

The culture that makes us afraid of the fat, the
floppy, the soft and sap-sweet, is the culture that kills
us. And the recovering anorexic is not only in a particularly good position to articulate these truths, she
is also, ironically, in a particularly good position, via
therapy, to treat the misogynist male. She understands
perhaps better than anyone the urge to whip and

dominate, to discipline and even delete the female form. I understand. I made my body a whitened bone, a pale blade. Like any real man, for years I lived with my fist and not my flesh. I was so hungry, but I could not risk the softness of surrender. I dreamt about letting down my guard, sitting at a table on which silver dishes steamed, and ingesting colors. Orange carrots, the soft wombs of tomatoes, the tangy dirt of a chocolate cake. But I couldn't dare, couldn't trust myself enough to let myself go. My head was empty except for the willpower that drove me on and the fear that I would fall through into life.

These were the memories that came to mind when I looked at Peter, so rigid in his chair, his face set against the seepage of any emotion that wasn't cruel or lewd, his skin so tattooed I couldn't have found a plain limb to touch if I had wanted to. He told me about forcing himself to rise before dawn each morning, working out two hours a day, jogging barefoot in the snow. He told me he made his girlfriend wear a "pussy ring," a tight gold band around her swelling sex. I nodded yes, having done the same to myself.

You could call my response countertransference. I call it building a bridge.

Of frayed rope and cracked sticks, a rickety bridge, no doubt. Nevertheless, I did not feel we were strangers, only estranged. Ours was a lonely therapy. The more deeply I went into it with him, the more difficult he became. Except for the brief stories he told me early on about his father's beatings, he absolutely refused to make himself vulnerable to me. Our therapy started to evolve so that I played a mostly silent role while he went on and on—endlessly, it seemed—about Joanne's anatomy, her "tight little box," the "six-hour plow" (I got sore just thinking about that), her sagless "bags," the nipple always hard in his hand. He spoke of split beavers and sucking dick ad nauseam.

"What about me?" I wanted to say to him. "Does it occur to you that I am a woman here, that you just might be *offending* me?" And beneath that, another, smaller voice was crying, "What about me; am I not also attractive, do I not measure up to your standards; why not?"

I began to realize our sessions were a lot like porn, in which I, the silent subject, absorbed his fantasies, and, in my featurelessness, reflected them back to him so that we both remained trapped in unalterable images of bondage. Peter let me know clearly what my role in our relationship was, by shifting impatiently whenever I spoke, by the quick brushing motions he made with his hands as though to sweep away my words, by interrupting me and then explod-

ing in a tyrannical temper if I asserted my right to finish my own sentence.

"Quiet!" he once roared at me, and I, like a little
girl, sank back down in my seat and felt darkness
grow up around me. At other times, I imagined
myself in sequins, my crotch sprayed silver, as I, nude,
gyrated to the beat of his voice.

"I wonder if you ever think," I finally burst out to
him one day, trying to chase images of leopard skins
and loincloths from my head as I spoke, "that I might
be uncomfortable with your sexual talk, with the, uh,
kinds of expressions you use."

"But you're a shrink," Peter said to me. "That's
what you're here for, to listen to my expressions.
That's your whole job."

"First of all," I said, "my whole job is not simply to
sit and listen, but to go with you as your co-worker,
co-discoverer, into the issues that make your life difficult, so we can work them out *together*. And second
of all" (I felt a snarl creep into my voice), "not even in
my office am I just a shrink. I am also a woman, and
the way you talk about my gender disgusts me." I
wanted to reach out and slap him, see my palm's tiny
but powerful print on his white cheek.

"I wouldn't talk like that to a woman I was trying
to make it with. But you're not supposed to—"

"Supposed to what?"

Peter looked uncomfortable. Halle-fuckin-lujah, I thought. I imagined I saw the colors on his Indian-princess tattoo start to blur and bleed.

"Supposed to mind," he said.

"Surprise," I said. "I mind." Tapping the side of my head: "I have a mind."

Peter looked up at me, his expression confused. My face felt all red. For one moment then, our masks dropped away. The static stereotypes shifted, crumbled. I could tell by the way Peter was looking at me that he was, for maybe the first time, considering me not as a function but as a feeling. I smiled at him.

He nodded, hello.

Shortly after this encounter Peter left the state for six weeks to do a series of carpentry jobs in Arizona. During the time he was away I found myself thinking of him in the desert, in the small Indian towns with the clumps of blowing tumbleweed; was he lonely? Lost? I thought of him running his hands over the contours of rock, feeling within it the craggy father face; in my imagination he was there, with long blond planks of wood, which, as he held them, turned to hanks of soft hair in his hands.

He returned to therapy in late May, deep spring in the North, the rose's red claw beginning to open. It was raining the day we resumed our sessions, and he stepped into my office soaking wet, beaded eyelashes, T-shirt stuck to his chest so the two tiny thorns of his nipples showed. His thick wavy hair was plastered down on a suddenly small skull; his shorts clung to buttocks I, for the first time, recognized as bony.

When I was a child I had a Shih Tzu dog, a high-blown, hairy canine with a fierce temper. I still have a small pale scar on my knee where he tore out a hunk of my six-year-old skin. The first time my mother gave the dog a bath is etched in my memory as one of the most remarkable metamorphoses I've witnessed in my lifetime. She dunked him, struggling, into a tub of water, and he came up, fluffed hair now wet as a second skin, a thin little animal with the tracings of bone visible beneath his hide. Even his tail, that gorgeous caramel-colored flare of fur, was no more than a piece of old raveled rope hanging over a pitifully pink naked anus.

Peter shivered in the air-conditioned building and goose bumps, like tiny buds, appeared all over his tattoos. I stared because I had never seen so much spontaneous movement on Peter's body before, any evidence that he wasn't willing, controlling. *Wet Peter,* I thought, *I like you.*

So it was a moment before I saw his expression. His eyes were hooded with exhaustion, ringed by blue, his face, untouched by the southern sun, too pale. He slumped down in his seat, looked at his lap.

"I was going to call you," he said, his voice low. I had never heard him use that voice before, a raw tone that brought to my mind a sapling branch stripped of its bark, and his voice elicited, for the first time, something gentle and even aching in me.

"What happened?" I asked.

"She left me," Peter said. He shook his head. "Just like that." He snapped his fingers in the air.

I was torn, surprised. I felt glad for Joanne. I had often worried about her safety with Peter, especially when he told me stories about shoving her, punching her, once even hauling her toward an open second-story window. I was glad she had finally gathered the courage to strike out on her own—this woman I had never met. But Peter looked awful.

"I came back from Arizona—the closets are empty, her picture's gone, not even a note. I called her at her parents' and she says it's completely finished. Gonzo. But I'm chasing her; I'm running after her like some goddamn desperate dog." Peter shook his head in confusion. "Me," he said, "making a fool of myself, phoning her ten, twenty times a day, bawling in her ear, but she's just wood. It doesn't matter what I do."

"It doesn't matter what you do," I said. "Tell me more about that."

"I've never not been able to convince someone, to force someone if I needed to, into doing what I wanted. But I've been trying every ploy with this cunt for the past week and I'm—"

"What? You're what?"

"Helpless." His mouth was a bitter line of tension, but his eyes were wet.

"I think that's what upsets you most about Joanne's leaving. That you have no control, that you feel helpless to get her back."

To my surprise, Peter nodded in agreement. His own pain had made him flexible, open to vision and suggestion. I also wondered if, having seen me step out of my stereotype in our previous meeting, he now felt freer to step out of his.

"I've never, *never* felt this way before. I've been stabbed in the neck, but this is way worse. I'm afraid to go home. I'm afraid to be alone. I didn't know I could ever have pain like this. How can it be so bad? *This is not me.*"

"But it is you, only a part of you you've managed, until now, to ignore."

For the first time in six months of treatment, I think we really talked. We exchanged. He had opened himself to me with his honest questions. Pain almost always does this, its intensity, like a hot spray, clearing away the dirt of denial. Perhaps this is one reason why, after we cry, we feel cleansed.

During this session, when Peter asked why and trembled, he brought up a lot of historical material, his relationship with his father, moments of abandonment, and all of this was important, but even more so was the intimacy now building between us, our voices low, our expressions intent, not masked. It was clear to me, as I think it was to Peter, that an admission of his own helplessness was an admission of his own humanity—the two were inextricably bound, and only from these could real talk, real touch, grow. "I feel we got something accomplished in this session," Peter said, "but I'm not sure what or how."

"I think it's that we really connected," I said. "I felt much closer to you in this session than I have before. I know you're really terrified of your own openness, or weakness even, because you're afraid of being taken advantage of, but as far as I'm concerned, it's just the opposite. Your willingness to finally talk about your own pain lets me see how complicated, and I guess colorful, you really are."

Peter smiled. "Of course," he said. "I'm no simple Joe Schmoe. I'm quite a case, huh?" He looked at me proudly, thumped on his chest.

We laughed a little, and then the hour was up.

. . .

The next few weeks brought some changes in Peter. He found himself facing an emotion he could not defend himself against. No amount of swearing or swaggering could express mourning. The pain of Joanne's leaving so suddenly broke his shield with an intensity neither of us had anticipated and brought up memories for him, as though, by going into a red wound, he had touched a new layer of his life. I was reminded of being in the Caribbean as a little girl and seeing, after a violent, sobbing storm, a school of dead sharks washed up on the beach, the silver bodies, surprisingly lovely, laid out on the sand. Peter remembered touching his father's face once when the man was sleeping, pedaling his bike to a pond in the summer, finding, one winter, a squirrel with something yellow dripping from its mouth, as something yellow was now dripping from his, some courage curdled and soured, some sadness. But to me he was not sour at all. The texture of our sessions altered. In his admission of pain he was now naked; he had pressed himself against me and I wanted to celebrate, not violate, this stance.

I was drawn to Peter now and I told him so, told him that for six months I had seen only a posture, and now I was seeing a person, and this person was brave.

"Brave?" Peter said to me. "I can't believe what a wreck I am. I can't believe that I'm falling apart over some bitch. You call that brave?"

"You're a lot braver now than you were before," I said, "when you were too scared to face your own soul. To me," I said, "and these are just my own values, but to me, as a woman, I think of a man as someone who is strong enough to experience himself, not afraid of taking voyages, instead of standing stuck in a block of cement."

I think he was a little grateful to me for saying that, for telling him I found him masculine in the moments he considered his worst.

For the next few weeks Peter ricocheted between two ways of being. Outside of therapy he was his usual hostile and inappropriate self, fighting with people, threatening Joanne over the phone. But within the office, the combination of his now-surfaced suffering and the deepening level of trust between us made him open. In some moments I think I saw his real face, the flow of emotion across it like wind working on sand. Those days, early summer, the sounds of the city streets drifting up to us—the millions of languages of the modern world, the occasional roar of an airplane in its angle of ascent—we discussed ancient myths and fairy tales, specifically the voyage of the archetypal hero who must leave his father's structured, cool castle and step into the messy wreckage of woods, the rotting leaves, in order to find a solid and secure authority within himself. It was crucial for Peter to be able to relate his painful journey to a grand mythic structure, to see that the rotting leaves of his soul were part of a socially sanctioned male odyssey. And I, well, I grew to love him and love the strength in his slow surrender.

It is June, I am twenty-one years old, I have not yet met Peter. I am just out of college. I weigh eighty-eight pounds. The heat of this month is thick as wet angora; the waxy leaves on the trees droop. When I look out my bedroom window I can see the tulips; they are the most trusting beings, they with their throats always open, their long gold tongues hanging out. Nothing bad happens to them; the sun doesn't rape them; they don't gag on the rain.

This day is really many months. I watch the world. I watch the natural cycle of things. Cliché as it may be, this is what cures me.

There comes a moment when recovery is religious, when the person says, "All right. I will have faith. I will lay down my sword and shield and see what the world works in me."

It is a dangerous thing for us, we people who grow up suckling the steel nipples of this country's missiles, men who think living in the world is living in a war, women who think their bodies are Molotov cocktails that must be detonated, destroyed, before they are munched up by their own metabolisms. What symbols do we have of safety?

I look away from my bedroom window and go downstairs, out onto the porch. Someone has set a table for me, my sister or an angel, I don't know. Sliced strawberries lie like the tongues of maidens on a platter. Wedges of cheese and bread. I put food in my mouth; for the first time in years I swallow the softness of ice cream. I want to see if my body will blow up in fatness with this slow animal stupidity swelling in my stomach. It doesn't. Letting down my guard, opening my many mouths, does not bring about the ruin, the rape I had feared. On the contrary. Food brings vitality back to me. I feel my hair take on sheen, grow longer, as though new stalks of thought are springing from my brain. My brain, now nourished, thinks in colors instead of calories. I can run harder; my eyes are moist enough to cry. It takes me years to learn this, but in my memory just a day goes by. A sun sets. Food is fuel, the weakness that makes us want it our greatest strength.

Peter started to taste—styles, voices, times. He reported allowing himself to sleep late one morning, waking to a room where light quivered on the walls. He started going out some nights without his leather vest or black boots, tried kissing a woman on the neck and "going no farther." He brought wood home with him at the end of working days, stayed up late making small objects without any obvious function— a box, a mobile, a chiseled plaque. It turned out he was good not only at nailing things together, but also at carving out designs, the chisel nuzzling slowly into the pine, yellow shavings like the rinds of lemons littered around him.

One day he came to session and told me he had met a woman—Lucky—with whom he thought he could fall in love, "if only I could get over Joanne."

"The other problem," Peter said, "is that she's the greatest person but she's heavy, maybe thirty pounds overweight. I've never made it with a fat woman before. You know me—I'm used to perfect curves, thighs I can grab a hold of, someone I can flip like a doll." He gave me one of his lewd Peter smiles.

I was enchanted by the idea of Peter with a fat woman, although, as often happens in therapy, his changes would begin to frighten him, and he would eventually retreat back into his shell, which was, nevertheless, not nearly as brittle as before. This leads me to believe that even the most entrenched personality disorder is open to change. And I had seen enough of him changed, naked, to imagine how his body would be within a fat woman's arms. I imagined her rocking him and him kissing her face and mouth. I could not help but see her spread legs on a bed, and he, a little cowed by the sight of so much, trying to touch her, first with his fingers, then with his penis, allowing himself entry into the many layers of her life; with his penis he brushes her uterus, goes up gently past her hip, until at last he touches the curved rib bone, the hard male bone, taken a long time ago from the man, buried and found only in the full woman's body.

SOME KIND
OF CLEANSING

1

No one knows for sure why the schizophrenic has such a hard time with words, why so little of his language makes sense. Ask him how the weather is and he might tell you, *Frogs be flying a green way.* Ask him about the Yankees game he stares at on the TV screen and he could well respond, *Pastimes that glump up are good.* Is this mumbo jumbo due to a dysfunction of the parictal lobe, that crescent of gray matter in the center of our skulls, or to some other kind of neuronal collapse? Or is it due to the schizophrenic's mother, who, early on, tongue-tied him with an overbearing love? People cannot definitively say. And we cannot go to the sources themselves, the actual schizophrenics, because they will babble or write a reason so jumbled it will hurt our own heads. I touch my own head, feel its spherical shape, feel the pulse of my voice pass from axon to dendrite and finally emerge from my mouth in blessed sentences. I watch as I press a series of separate keys on this computer and up through the gas plasma screen drifts a story for you. And for me. In this way we join. The ability to use words, to tell a story, is so central to having human relationships that I find myself wondering how someone with schizophrenic illness survives the loss. When the men I work with weep or scream or clench their hands, I think they are mourning their muteness. There's frustration on their faces. As they attempt to talk, I sometimes try to catch glimpses of their tongues, expecting to see not the limber red scalpel that shapes a sentence, but a flapping gray thing, loose and dead.

I remember not knowing language very well. I keep this memory close to me as I work with schizophrenic illness because it's a tiny door by which I might enter that silent or scrambled world. I was six. I was in kindergarten, and boggy May air drifted through the open classroom windows. Outside, bees zipped from white hive to hedge and flowers pumped out of the earth. I was happy. My teacher, Miss Austen, picked up a piece of chalk and onto the board put F-A-T C-A-T. "Read," Miss Austen said, stepping back and waiting.

In my memory then, we were standing behind our desks. Perhaps we were really sitting, but I recall, suddenly, the clench of my calves, a stiffening in the sockets of my knees. I was just learning to read, and still so unsure of how to do it, wobbling along the spines of sentences as I would later wobble on the backs of horses, trying to keep both balance and grace. "Read," Miss Austen said again, and I wanted to read but I couldn't. I stared at the letters on the board. I knew each individual shape; that arch was an *A;* that teacup on its side a *C.* But I couldn't put the letters together. "EFFFF," I spluttered, "ahhhhh," and then "tee tee tee." It bothered me. No, it more than bothered me; it scared me. I couldn't read! How quickly the world breaks down, sense scrambles. I stared at the dashes between the letters. The long white light of the room winced like a migraine. "FFFF—AAAA—T; FAT! And then with that sudden twist of understanding came CAT! and onto the blackboard of my mind shimmied a deliciously fat cat, butter-colored and whiskered, her long tail linking around me as she purred the world back to being.

I know just a little bit, oh just a tiny bit of the fear that comes from a world without sensible words. I know it from my memory of that kindergarten classroom and then I know it again from watching Joseph D'Agostino on the residential unit for chronic schizophrenics where I work. Of all the tongue-tied schizophrenics I know, he stands out for me as an effigy of such suffering. Joseph is forty-six years old. He has a mangy black beard in which lice like to live, and on some days he wears a floppy bow tie, on other days an army helmet and a green shirt with fake medals of honor dangling from the pockets. Although he claims to have crouched in the foxholes of World War I and sloshed through the jungles of Vietnam, Joseph, in actuality, has never been to war in the way we know it. The terrors live within him; the bombs are bursts of dopamine that sting the raw ravines of his brain.

I encountered Joseph—with whom I was to do individual therapy—during my first week on the ward. He was also one of the six men in my group, which had just gathered for the first time. I was slowly starting to adjust to the place, to the long scrubbed corridors and the drone of the TV perched high in a corner of the kitchen. To the patients who, in their free time, sat on the deck smoking endless packs of cigarettes and lecturing to invisible students. The ward was, of course, bizarre, the banal noise of daytime TV game shows mixed in with shrieks and fantastic tales about harems of wives who climbed through windows each night. The ward manager's name was Eddie Harrington, but the patients, for a reason no one knew, called him Eddie Dream. He was an old white-haired man, bent in his back and legs, who stuck placard reminders all around the unit:

EDDIE DREAM SAYS:
PLEASE DISPOSE OF ALL CIGARETTES IN THE ASHTRAYS

EDDIE DREAM SAYS:
CLEAN UP THE DECK BY SEVEN PLEASE

IF YOU'RE NOT OUT OF BED BY EIGHT-THIRTY BOYS
I WILL WRITE YOU UP
—EDDIE DREAM

And it was in this strange world of smoke and shrieks and magic messages that I first met Joseph. He was unlike the other patients. He did not sit in the common room or the kitchen watching endless hours of TV or staring into space. Instead, Joseph passed his days in the spare bedroom across from the staff office, where there was just an unmade cot and a plain desk surrounded by beige walls. The blinds in that room were always drawn, and a shadeless lamp burned in one corner. When I first met Joseph, he, or someone, had draped a handkerchief over the bulb so the room had a reddish glow, and Joseph was in the midst of this disturbing light, bunched in a ball at the desk, holding a pencil and scribbling furiously into a Harvard University notebook. I would soon learn that, unlike his fantasies of Vietnam and World War One, Joseph had once really gone to a school like Harvard and his wish to go back there was tangled up with his wish for a mind that could make well-ordered words.

But there was nothing well ordered about this man. Torn-up napkins, scraps of paper, tattered bits of notebook, lay at Joseph's feet. There was drool in his beard. "Hello," he muttered, glancing up at me as I stood in the doorway's entrance, and then he went right back to his consuming task. Curious and also frightened, I crept forward into that room. I wanted to see what it was he was doing, what work commanded so much of his attention. At the same time, though, stepping into that room felt like stepping into someplace far away, an isolated island, an underwater world where the sun filters down to you in weak streaks you cannot reach. I was afraid the door might slam behind me, an invisible lock would click us closed. I went anyway.

Close to him, I peered over his shoulder. His handwriting was terrible; the drugs he was taking made his whole body shake, so the letters tilted and crashed, but in between the shards I could make out a sentence that said, "Jesus Christ came into the sanctuary for a past time where pregnant girls meant to effigure an elder statesman." Drip went some drool.

"You see," he said, jabbing his finger at a clot of wet words. "You see how the dictionary measures it? I am trying to measure it. I wish with a dowager's meaning that I could separate it, that I could read and write again. I can't except to say that to suck is to suck is to sssuck a donkey's dick!"

And with that he shot up out of his chair so fast I leapt back. He towered over me, and had huge blundering feet in cracked black shoes. His face was like his sentences, the features jammed on wrong, a nose too far to the left, a bumpy forehead. His eyes swung around the room, noticing everything but me, and then he snatched up his pages again, lifted them close to his face, as though proximity might bring meaning. "Where where?" he whispered, and I heard terror in his voice. I saw the shaking of his limbs was not just drug-induced; it came from fear as well. "I don't know what I mean," he said, scanning his sentences, and that's when I remembered the kindergarten classroom, trying to pry sense out of letters slashed separate by white marks. Without language we are lost.

"My head," he said, "has been pocked up by needles. Knives. Fat-charged electrons. Peck Peck."

"My name is Lauren," I said softly. "I will be your new therapist."

He put the pages back down, turned toward me.

"Oh," he said. "I see. I am Joseph D'Agostino, of the Teddy Bear Lounge."

He smiled then, lips parting over a set of gleaming front teeth like white tablets. I thought of the tablets God handed down to the Sinai, on them written the commandments that made some lives sane. Perhaps somewhere in this crazy man were some sensible sentences, some coherent stories. Perhaps we would find them, and soothe his terrors. My heart calmed.

"Nice to meet you," I said.

"And to you," he said, "I will give a B with two plus three pluses." In goodwill then, he extended his arm toward me, and it was a second before I realized that this was not his hand I was shaking, nor his finger, but the pencil.

He was a man of great goodwill, but also a terribly sad and frustrated person. Joseph wrote with a vengeance, with the sort of compulsion that might have made him an artist had he possessed the ability to organize his thoughts. In the middle of dinner he might grab hold of a napkin and fire a stream of nonsensical words onto it. When staff cleaned up his room they found rolled-up bits of paper under his pillow. In the office they unfolded the papers and saw sentences that included descriptions of iguana eggs set side by side with remarks about kitchen plates. Schizophrenia is so many things, such a messy pile of symptoms, but if there's one common thread that runs through the disorder it is that of disorganization. Psychologists call this phenomenon *overinclusion,* and it means that the schizophrenic patient lacks the capacity to put information into appropriate categories. Give the schizophrenic the task of sorting objects into piles, and he or she will get completely confused. Into the cup pile will also go straws and pen caps, the dead ant on the floor. Into the picture pile will go book jackets and pillowcases, a coffee mug, a cuckoo clock. "I must take in the whole room," one schizophrenic patient lamented during just such an experiment. Overinclusion is maddening, no pun intended. Probably because he was sensitive and smart, Joseph seemed to know he mushed the whole world together, seemed to know his thoughts blurred and bled. ("I am trying to measure it. I wish with the dowager's meaning that I could separate it, that I could read and write again.") He was my patient. And I have always thought his efforts to create an organized written account, to tease the twistedness apart, were heroic and poignant.

. . .

And irritating too, for both of us. His linguistic chaos caused him not only fear but also frustration. I, for my part, felt frustrated because he was not an easy person to know, or, in the parlance of psychology, "to engage in treatment." I could not connect with Joseph in a way that felt satisfying. For instance, whenever I approached him in the hall, hoping to make some kind of conversation, he would back away, then dart forward, jerking his head like a rooster. He would snatch a pen from his shirt pocket and begin writing on whatever surface he could find. But his words did little to bring us together. While we usually think of language as a series of strings between me and you, drawing us close in communion, with Joseph words were a wall.

And on Joseph's part, the frustration seemed to have something to do with knowing he was not making any sense and being helpless to alter that fact. Joseph was a smart man. His I.Q. scores from the eighth grade, before he got ill, show him to have once had a verbal aptitude in the superior range. Surely one would feel the smack of such a loss. Retested four years ago, Joseph's verbal I.Q. score was now subnormal, indicating retardation. He had a keenness of perception, though, a full-fledged awareness of missing things. The unit was located across from a high school, and every afternoon Joseph stood at the common-room window, watching with what looked like longing as kids with notebooks, kids with neatly printed papers they'd done on their own, poured out the doors. "Joseph," I might call at such moments. "Joseph, Joseph, it's time for a snack, it's time for group," but he would hardly ever answer. Other times I saw him press his pencil harder and harder onto the page, his whole body tight with tension, and still no sense emerging.

"What is it like?" I asked him one day, "Joseph, what is it like to be so confused about words?"

I knew my question was ridiculously and perhaps cruelly direct, but I wanted to know, and besides, with such a patient, I reasoned, the fewer fripperies surrounding a sentence the better.

We were sitting in the spare bedroom again, the door open and staff bustling up and down the corridor outside. "It is like," he said to me slowly, and I got the impression he was swimming deep within himself for the answer, "it is like . . . being trapped inside the dragon."

This was maybe the first cogent thing he had ever said to me—the first small story he had ever told—and because stories form pictures, I saw a boy in the red belly of a dragon, a boy pressing his eyes against scaly inner skin and finding nothing.

He stared steadily at me, and for a moment we were together. "I have," he said, speaking very softly, "a special book." He looked down at the desk, traced the wood's grain with one finger, and then his body started to shake. "Excellence, my excellence," he said. "A special book."

"Let me see," I said.

He fished about in one of the desk's drawers and pulled out several large sheets of brown paper rolled into a scroll, which he slowly, with shaking hands, unfurled for me. At the top of the first sheet I saw written, in bold tilting letters, ALPHABETS AND LINGUAGELES OF THE WHOLE WORLD. Later on, when reading Dr. Susan Baur's and other psychologists' descriptions of mad writers, I would learn that such scrolls and booklets are not that uncommon, nor the long lists of squished and stuttering words comprising them. At the time, though, I was half shocked, half enchanted. "Che che che Chinese," Joseph spluttered. "My Greek." And sure enough, as his finger moved down the lines of his writing, I saw he had compiled these words with what looked like confused attempts at translations beside them. "Kimereah," he had written, and then, "Kelesquelia in Spanish?? Egyptian Chro—mera?"

"Beast," he had written, and beneath it, "Francaise feast. Chinese dragonlimla. Which one is true???"

And as my eyes moved across the length of this scroll, I thought of the Torah I'd studied as a young girl, the rabbi lifting it with reverence from its silver arc, the laws scripted inside, written and rewritten, debated and decoded over centuries of time in the quest to understand.

I moved to the next sheet. "Illusionary," Joseph had written there.

> To dream
> along the eddie
> old man and comparisions in the tabernacle
> my name is Joseph Hpesoj
> A PRINCETON PERSON
> YES NO YES

"A special book," I said, "of languages and words. What do the words mean, Joseph?"

He looked at what he'd written, turned the pages over and over, traced the letters slowly, sadly. He shrugged. "Can't explain," he said, and his voice was full of defeat. And then he flipped to the last piece of paper, where, in large block letters, surrounded with drawings of dove-shaped wings, Joseph had written:

OH THAT I COULD GO TO THE SKY
WHERE I MIGHT FIND A CLEAR KNOWING

I went home that night and woke up late to a pitch-dark room. I had had a bad dream, I think. My shades were drawn and it was that hour well before dawn where the blackness is so thick it stifles shapes. I waited then, heart paddling, for a headlight to sweep along the wall, white as a dove's wing, showing me the place where I slept—clothes heaped on the floor, the books on my shelves, the cherry-wood trunk—these things I could not see that formed the language of my life.

Before he got sick, Joseph lived out much of his life in Boston's North End, that small Italian community crammed into one corner of the city. As a neighborhood, the North End is known for its coherence; families stay together, oftentimes great aunts and grandparents living in the same apartments as their younger offspring. Joseph's upbringing was that way. I didn't learn these details from him, of course, but from his sister, Vickie, who sometimes came to visit him, and from the voluminous hospital charts kept in the locked cabinet of the staff room.

I can easily picture the house where he grew up, easily picture the stores with their striped awnings and the alley that ran beneath his bedroom window. I can imagine his Mediterranean grandmother from whose lips came English, Italian, or French, depending on her mood. Joseph grew up in a multi-tongued family, grew up in a rich linguistic sea where words and stories were well stocked.

Not all of the stories were verbal. Joseph's father, Salvatore, was a proud and domineering man who had come to this country with the intention of making a name for himself. That he did. While alive, he owned the most prominent Italian restaurant in town. It still exists today, famous for its pasta now sold in supermarkets across the country. All of the family— Joseph's older brothers and younger sister, the parents and the grandparents—were involved in the restaurant, all helped make meals that were exquisitely balanced among delicate beginnings, satisfying middles, and conclusive ends. Vickie described the father's relentless pride in appearances, the painstaking detail that went into peeling shrimp for the appetizers, the cheese melted to a specific softness with just the right amount of brown around its drooping edges. The family told stories not just through words, but through food as well—these elaborate meals they cooked in the restaurant's kitchen.

As a boy, Joseph had participated in the cooking. He had been bright-eyed and intelligent and had, so Vickie informed me, adored the names of exotic ingredients, letting them linger on his tongue as though the sounds themselves were spiced. "Let's sprinkle in some

pap-a-r-ika," the five-year-old Joseph would say.
"Let's try some nutmeg." Early on, I think, he knew
the poetry in certain words, the way any activity could
become a story, even a meal, or a kitchen where a family minced and sliced—steaks on the plate and long
strings of dried tomatoes tying up the tale.

It was a life rich in detail, in the sensual stuff that
makes up romance, in the structures that form a son-
net. The pain, if there was any, must have had something to do with the father's tyrannical nature, how
he threatened to smack with the wooden spoon
should his children loaf in his kitchen, how he pressed
them to dress well, to sashay onto the dining-room
floor each Saturday evening and, tiny maître d's, snap
open the white linen napkins folded like swans on top
of the table. I only imagine this, though. I only glean
hints of this from lines in hospital charts that describe
the father as "stern and uncommunicative. Salvatore
D'Agostino appears to expect a lot from his son."

And this son Joseph, for a while he lived up to the
expectations. He lilted the names of spices and was
famous in his family, in his whole neighborhood, for
his brains. No one in the family had ever gone to college. Everyone knew Joseph would. His mother,
whom he loved to distraction, knew he would. I picture her as a dark-haired lady with the smell of
Europe still on her skin, a mother who doted on her

son with the kind of attention that leads to anxiety. ("Joseph and Mom were so close," Vickie informed me. "She thought he was the sweetest and the smartest. He was her great pride.")

In the sixth grade, Joseph took a test to get into one of Boston's exam schools, and from the seventh grade on he attended Boston Latin, where he graduated third in his class. ("He wanted to be a social psychologist or a novelist. We didn't have any doubts about that. And, no, even when I look back on it now, knowing everything that's happened to him, I can't find any evidence of his illness coming on.")

Was he good-looking? Popular? Did he have a girlfriend? None of this is mentioned in his sister's story of Joseph's childhood and adolescent days. We all have ways we brand ourselves, special knacks we come to fondle as central to our being. With Joseph, the knack was clearly connected to smarts, the ability to create and articulate order. Thus, I saw his schizophrenic writing not so much as an attempt to contain anxiety but, rather, as an attempt to retrieve certain crucial aspects of his identity that were decimated by his disease.

Fall 1966, and recruiters were coming to the exam schools, sending out letters to candidates they wanted to court. Some kids got invitations to apply based on athletic abilities; Joseph, so the sister told me, was recruited for his academic performance, outstanding PSAT scores and a 3.9 GPA. Each semester he brought his report cards home, and each semester his father held them up to the light as store managers hold up one-hundred-dollar bills, checking as to their veracity before enfolding them in their tills. All of Joseph's grades went into the family till, but I don't believe every bit of love revolved around performance. The mother's love, it seems, was something larger, something lusher. He was her child, born from her belly. She saw her face in his. At night, before he dropped off to sleep, the mother would creep into Joseph's bedroom, stroke his sleek black hair, and sing that boy to sleep.

He applied and was accepted to Princeton, the first child in his immigrant family to go off to college. I do not know how he felt, with such a load of expectations on his back. I do not know if the duffel bags he carried off that first semester were weighted more with the family's hopes than with his clothes. Grandmothers, aunts, siblings, neighbors, saw him off at the bus terminal. And it must have seemed like a slash, like a cruel sort of severance, one moment lodged in the tiny nest of some city, the next moment released into the ivy air, facing a sprawling green campus and kids who owned their own cars. He would be a literary critic, a social psychologist. He would pronounce the spices of these subjects perfectly.

Instead, four weeks into that first semester at Princeton, he started to stare at things and laugh. ("In one class, the professor told us, he kept flapping his hand in front of his face, over and over again.") By the eighth week he was smoking several joints a day and not coming out of his room. He got into a fight with a dorm mate and put his fist through a window. Just before Christmas, when the ivy had fallen, stripped veins clinging to the sides of buildings, he confided to a friend that there were microphones hidden inside the stems.

He left on a bus for Christmas break. I wonder what he saw, driving back through the countryside, dry clouds scraping the sky. I feel great fear for him at this point in our story. I think about the brown blades of winter in the barren fields, maybe the first snow starting to fall, each flake, in his eyes, articulated to the point of pain, white prongs, a dazzle of frozen lace.

Was he looking for warmth, for a way to connect with a world that had suddenly slipped from him? Is that why, once home, he walked into his family's living room and, in front of mother, father, aunts, unbuckled his pants and exposed himself? "Look at me," he wailed, tugging at his penis. Salvatore leapt up and slapped him. The mother wept. His report card came a few days later, a slew of D's and F's.

He never went back to Princeton. For a long time after that he did not go out of the North End at all. He was overcome by delusions and hallucinations, and his speech deteriorated. His clothes got grungy and he would tramp home at two A.M. smelling of booze and back alleys. The family sought professional help, frequently had him hospitalized, but nothing worked. Years passed. Horrified, the father shunned him, would not allow this disheveled son into the restaurant. The mother drew even closer to him, bathing her boy, combing his matted hair, and dressing him in a neat black suit to wear to the father's funeral when Salvatore finally passed away. After that, with the other children grown and gone, the oldest son now running the restaurant, just Joseph and his mother lived together, she doing everything for him while he paced and ranted in his room. He lost the ability to wash his hair, make a meal. Down in the kitchen, she fried eggs for him, smooth white globes of wholeness she would crack against the side of a pan, watch the shocking yellow innards spill, sizzle.

After Joseph's mother died and there was no one to take care of him, the sister and brother placed him here, in this inner-city residential unit located four trolley stops from the North End. Because the unit is open, the men—unless they are suicidal—can come and go as they please, without escort. Without escort, then, Joseph, in between groups and individual therapy, often likes to ride the trolley back to his old neighborhood. Perhaps he even goes to the house where he once lived, sees in the windowpane's reflection the fragile face of his mother, the triumphant white swans floating on his father's tables. At work, when I look at him sitting in that spare bedroom, I try to imagine who he could have been. I focus on his chapped wet mouth, and in my mind I sculpt its lines smooth. I bend over and blow the duff from his fogged eyes. For me, it is hard to match the Joseph I now know—the frustrated, word-bound man—with the bright boy who so loved language, who, with a Boston Latin pencil, could shape letters into moving compositions.

A few days ago, Eddie Dream repaved the sidewalk outside of the unit. He poured wet concrete out of a barrel, smoothed it over with a trowel, and then hung up one of his famous signs:

EDDIE DREAM SAYS THE CONCRETE IS WET BOYS
USE THE BACK WAY

But Joseph, either because he couldn't read the sign, so wrapped up in a mad world was he, or because he didn't want to obey the sign from some defiance, trudged out there anyway. I think he saw a moment where he could make his mark. Army helmet strapped on, black combat boots, medals of honor glinting in the fall sun, he tromped onto the spongy surface, never once looking down, writing his way across that tiny world. No one knew until it was too late, and the concrete had dried, and there were his footprints, the letters of Joseph, a solid signature of self for all to see.

2

There is a name for Joseph's compulsive writing—*hypergraphia*. A syndrome usually found in patients with temporal-lobe epilepsy, hypergraphia also sometimes affects the mentally ill, causing in its sufferers a compulsive need to write, whether or not the prose makes sense.

Some of the most startling and eloquent accounts of hypergraphia are recorded by Dr. Susan Baur, who in turn has drawn from an article by S. Waxman and N. Geschwind in a contemporary journal of neurology. Dr. Baur tells the story of a young woman named Yolanda, who created a dictionary of "autographs and forgeries," while Waxman and Geschwind tell a still more bizarre tale of a young secretary whom they treated for several months. Sitting at her typewriter, she found herself suddenly "beset by unexpected orgasms." Embarrassed, flustered, she would clench her legs and mouth closed and pretend to be busy at work while her private sexual storms buffeted her about. Roughly half an hour after these orgasmic episodes, she would, each time, enter a trance and, still sitting at her typewriter, unbeknownst to any of her office mates, produce pages and pages of mystical writings.

While I don't believe Joseph experienced such specific sexual pleasures prior to or during his bouts of writing, there was a distinctly libidinal feel to his epistolary activities, the feel of a man aching for release and return to wholeness, as orgasm releases us from our fractured skins and returns us to a greener world—the smell of childhood, apple skins spiraling from the blade of a mother's knife, noises rising up to the window where we sleep, the clacking of a trolley in a darkly draped Mediterranean house. We come to it.

But he couldn't come to it. Orgasm, like any artistic or ecstatic feat, requires the fine-tuning of concentration, the mind as a single beam. Joseph, in his writings, in all of his activities, was so hopelessly scattered. Like other schizophrenics, he suffered from overinclusion, so that his stories contained bits of everything that came to nothing. Sometimes his sentences were so broad they spanned eons of time, as in: "Wind moving the grass where daddy rooster goes licking the skyscraper. I once rode up to the top and looked way down. Hi!" But Joseph's tendency toward overinclusion showed itself best in the way he packed for a camping trip Eddie Dream took the boys on late in August, about a year after I'd started on the unit. Going away for only two days, Joseph took it upon himself to pack five suitcases, four duffel bags, and a tower of crates. He brought all of his blankets, every pair of shoes, the pillows on his bed, the lightbulbs from the lamp, a fan, a hammer, a hole puncher, and two quarts of antifreeze. He appeared in front of the van with all of this stuff, and it took staff two hours to return the excess, marching up and down the unit's stairs.

How can you understand and connect to a man through whom the whole world sweeps and speaks, and how can that man understand and connect to you? That was the question informing my therapy with Joseph. Despite the plethora of words, ours was a silent journey, static everywhere we turned. If I tried to get him to put down his pencil and speak with me, he would moan and pick it back up again. If I asked him to write me how he was feeling, he produced a tome of chaos. Why was he doing this? Was his hypergraphia some mere neurological twitch, or a way to contain anxiety, or, what I most believed, a desperate and perpetually failing plea to become what he once was, a storyteller, a social participant whose words would break the barrier of isolation and thrust him into community? That is what we all want our stories, however meager, to do. With Joseph it didn't work.

And because it didn't work, I found myself wondering about the specifics of his language problem, for understanding origins can sometimes lead to cures. Prior to the popularity of neuropsychology, his linguistic confusion would have probably been explained as the result of poor ego boundaries, an inability to separate unconscious from conscious thought, so it all poured together and out onto the page. Now there was probably some fashionable physiological explanation for his fractured writing skills, but the literature I consulted claimed only the vaguest speculations: possible lesions on the Wernicke's area of the cortex, shriveled frontal lobes sometimes observed in the brains of schizophrenics. However, nowhere could I find any conclusive answers, because the brain is so inconclusively understood, and schizophrenia, as a brain disease, is still mired in darkness. That is one reason I felt so lost with Joseph, I supposedly "the expert," with so little knowledge of what was going on, and on top of that, so little ability to help him with his language confusion. Sometimes I stared and stared at his sentences. And I could find within them half-formed ideas, a growing pattern of thought that aborted itself in messy clots. All of our sessions took place in that spare bedroom, he bent over the desk, I standing by his side, watching powerlessly as he, because of some undefined illness, wrote walls and walls of babel around his body.

Until at last, one day, frustrated by the hypergraphia that kept me so severed from him, I leaned forward, plucked up the pencil, and scrawled my way right onto his page.

"The church," Joseph had written in his tilted letters, "is where the peropper people go. Worms sleep inside of me, all clouds and test tubes."

"I once went to church," I wrote back in careful large script. "I was only six, and I remember seeing Jesus on a cross on the wall."

Joseph turned his head and looked up at me, his mouth agape. He stared at me holding his pencil, and then he swiveled himself slowly and peered at the page where I had put my writing next to his. The room got strangely silent. I waited to see what would happen. I had been trying to begin a correspondence, somehow cross into his space. My gesture didn't have quite the effect I'd hoped for. Joseph kept staring and staring at my sentences, his eyes widening. Instead of writing back, he uncurled one grimy index finger and started to stroke the letters, my plump o, the sophisticated shape of my s. I was reminded of the way some ladies will stroke diamonds on the jeweler's velvet trays or put pearls to their powdered cheeks, longing in every movement. My letters next to Joseph's, I then realized, were jewels to him, crafted shapes that gleamed with sense. He kept tracing and retracing them, as though through touch he might absorb their gifts. "You are a doctor," he murmured, still fingering the shapes. "Pretty pretty."

He looked up at me then. "I once could," he said. He stopped.

"Could what, Joseph?"

He set his mouth in a bitter line and shook his head. He went back to patting my sentences. "I once could," he said again. Sadness in his voice. "You went to school, Doctor," he said.

I nodded my head yes.

He saw me nod and raised his eyes again, squinting them as he studied my face. For a long time he peered at my face, and then, as though he were blind, he reached for my nose, my eyebrows. I let him. I was scared. Was this sexual? Maybe, but something more, too. He was studying me, studying my shape, like a man remembering something, finding his former self. Like a scientist who traces the grooves of a fossil in stone, feeling his whole history etched there, lost and found. Lost and found.

"Harvard," Joseph said. "Your school was Harvard."

And I nodded again, because he happened to be right.

He snatched away his hand then, shoved it between his knees. "Harvard," Joseph said. "Harvard Harvard Harvard." He chanted and rocked, the rocking motions strengthening and I, suddenly scared, wondering what I'd set off in him.

"I, too," he shouted.

"I know," I said.

"I, too!" he bellowed, and he leaned back over the page to fondle my letters. "Bloomsbury," he spit. "Bloomsbury in bedlam."

I think, in feeling my face and my phrases, he must have recalled with too much clarity the man he was going to be before illness came on. Because something changed in Joseph after that interaction, something intensified. For the next few days, and to everyone's surprise, he didn't write anything at all. His compulsion screeched to a halt as though a deeper grief were whispering inside, from someplace where there were no words. "I am worried about Joseph," Sophie said in staff meeting that Wednesday. "He's not eating and he seems more disorganized than ever."

The week passed. Joseph wandered the halls, his eyes rimmed with red. "Harvard Harvard," he started to mutter under his breath. He peered out the window of the common room hours before it was time for the summer-school classes to end, watching for the kids to pour out of the high school doors, and when a man wearing a Yale sweatshirt walked by, he banged on the glass. "*Veritas,*" he said to the air, and made a little bow. He attached so many medals of honor to his army shirt that he clanged when he walked. Eddie reported to us that Joseph sat up in bed all Sunday night, one arm raised in the air.

And then, on Monday morning, he brought his arm down. He knocked on the door of the staff room, where the other counselors and I were meeting. "*Guten morgen,*" Joseph chirped. He nodded decisively at all of us. "I am going back to school," he announced.

"School?" Sophie echoed. As a mental-health aide on the unit, she was, along with three other aides, responsible for the men's daily comings and goings. "What school? What do you mean, Joseph?"

"Harvard," Joseph said. "*Veritas.*"

And then, before we could respond, he was off, out the door, and he didn't return for the rest of the day.

"They wouldn't let me register," he announced at dinner that night. His appetite appeared to be back, though. He scooped up a mound of mashed potatoes and shoved them in his mouth. He slurped a can of Coke. "Excellence, my excellence. Tomorrow, MIT!"

And he was off the next day, searching MIT to register. His steps were lighter. He paused in the middle of the hall and, before dancing out the door, scribbled a mysterious message in the air.

"Oh, no," Sophie said. "It's one thing for him to go around Boston looking for a school, but what happens when he doesn't find a place that will let him in, and so he decides, like before, to take a trip up to Yale, or even farther away, like Stanford?"

Six years before, when he had first come onto the unit, Joseph had gotten a similar sort of idea in his head, and had run off, disappearing for three weeks. He was finally found by New Jersey State Police walking the highways near Princeton.

"So maybe we should head the whole thing off by finding a place in Boston for him to register," said Bill. "If he really wants to go back to school, should we stop him anyway?"

In staff meeting that day we discussed the pros and cons of helping Joseph enroll in school. On the pro side, enrollment would definitely be a boost to his shattered self-esteem, giving him the hope that he might be able to regain his lost language skills. For that is how we interpreted his desire for school, not as a random reach for prestige but as a deliberate effort to retrain his pen and paper. But, maybe even more important, if we could get him registered at a school in the area, we might be diverting a frantic escapade to an Ivy League somewhere across the country. On the con side, Joseph was so disorganized we didn't see how he could succeed in any academic system, no matter how basic. And failure might toss him into a final depression.

"Can you really see Joseph in a classroom?" Jen, another aide, asked. "What would everyone do? He's too weird."

"Weirdness isn't a good enough reason to stop him from getting, or at least trying to get, what he wants," Bill said. "And it's not like he's dangerous or lewd. He'd never hurt anyone. He doesn't scream or swear."

"Yeah, but he looks—"

"Look," said Sophie. She was a large woman with long black curls, strong in her speech. "Regardless of what we say or do, he's going to try it anyway. And if that's the case, then I want to at least be involved. I'd rather help him find some kind of community college in Boston than worry he'll run away to New Haven."

And that made sense to us. With misgivings, and because Joseph agitated for several weeks to go back to a university, we finally, with funding from the Massachusetts Rehabilitation Commission, helped him register for two courses at an open-admissions school known for the diversity of its students—Admiral's Hill Community College. Located in a rough section of Charlestown, this community college boasted "an acceptance of students from all walks of life, from all over the globe. English and non-English speakers, old and young, handicapped people of all persuasions, are welcome here." We hoped Joseph would be welcome. We were not at all convinced. He wouldn't sign releases allowing us to talk to the school about his particular disabilities. And he chose, not surprisingly, some of the most demanding courses in social psychology and creative writing, two disciplines based on narrative, its creation and interpretation. "You're sure about this, Joseph?" Sophie said to him in the staff room. She shook her head. "You're sure you want to take these courses? Why not something more *applicable*? Why not . . ." and we watched her scan the catalog, looking down the list of remedial courses.

"No!" Joseph said when we suggested basic computer skills. "No robots!" He charged out of the office. A done deal. No robots for him. Social psychology, creative writing, a return to an earlier dream.

The semester was starting in just a few days. It was early September now, the trees shading into vulnerable apricots, pale reds. The enormous sunflowers in the city gardens were bowing their tired heads. Walking in the Commons after work one day, I found a dead swan on the ground next to the pond. Wind lifted its white feathers, its slender throat outstretched. Everywhere I looked I saw something wounded or gone. For Joseph, this return to school was a celebration—a chance for him to learn to tell a story again—but I, all of the staff, felt him walking into treacherous territory. We saw him finally facing, on the blackboards of those classrooms, in the stares of the other students, the truth about his severed mind.

In the four days before classes started, Joseph stayed busy. He spent his entire Social Security disability check on a briefcase, a suit, a pair of shoes, and, finally, an Aladdin lunch box. On the Tuesday after Labor Day he came downstairs for breakfast scrubbed and shining, the first time in years. He sported a fresh white shirt, Italian leather loafers, and a corduroy coat, and carried a brown briefcase and the lunch box, full to bursting not with food but with his fake army medals.

He was going back to school, rejoining the community. His illness had resulted in the loss of language. The loss of language had cut him off not only from deep sources of self but also from his connections with others. Hoping to tell a story, hoping to create a text, Joseph, it seemed, was trying to reaffirm his own talents while also placing himself smack in the middle of our contemporary culture. Schizophrenia is so many things, has such a multiplicity of consequences, one of which is the removal of the sufferer from society. No longer able to tell stories we can understand, the schizophrenic is bumped to the borders of our world, where we toss so many other senseless things. That morning, as we watched him leave for his first class, as we—Sophie, Bill, Eddie Dream, and I—stood at the door and saw him trudge down the city hill, we were watching, I thought, a man tapping on trap doors, looking for reentry.

He reentered the unit at four o'clock each evening. Right from the start, he refused to answer our questions about how his school days went. Each morning, though, when he came down for breakfast, he looked just a little bit grungier than the morning before, and by the end of the fourth week, his briefcase was bulging with crumpled-up scraps of paper and the buoyancy in his step had vanished. "You're not handing those papers in to the teacher, are you, Joseph?" Sophie asked.

He hugged his briefcase to him and wouldn't reply. In the following days, he seemed, if it was possible, crazier than ever. He kept batting his eyes, as though trying to clear sharp specks from his vision. "Maybe we should get in touch with the teachers of his courses and let them know what the problem is, that he's handicapped," Bill suggested.

But when we asked Joseph again to sign the release of information that would enable us to break his confidentiality, he tore it up. "Scalpels!" he screamed. "Chips from the CIA!" He hurled the briefcase across the room and balls of paper spilled out of its pouches.

Later, after he'd gone to sleep, I examined the papers. Of course, on most of them were mad scribbles, but some of them were stories he had tried to write, stories marred by a teacher's red pen. As I had so many times before, I peered at his sentences and paragraphs and saw glimmers of coherence in some of them, half-uttered themes that bled away into chaos. How could I tease sense from the shambles? And the shambles themselves, they did have a kind of haunting poetry that, I suspected, was so unsatisfying to Joseph because he appeared to have no control over it. The man could, without quite meaning to, write a tilted e. e. cummings–type paragraph, but not a simple shopping list. An odd kind of curse, no doubt. And then I saw that one of the papers was a multiple-choice quiz from the social psychology class. The grade was an F. "You have to pick one," the teacher had written across the top of the paper, and, looking down the columns, I saw that Joseph, too much in love with the world—the man through whom the whole world sweeps and speaks—had circled every choice, all possibilities existing.

"Yes, I am failing," he said when we asked him the next morning.

"Do you want to stop? You can always stop."

"I want to stop failing," he said.

3

I thought about him a lot during those early-fall days. Sometimes it happens that a patient brings up your own pain, and you enter his story, swimming down deep into the mind's green waters. I felt a clot in my throat, something that wouldn't let language come. I remembered times when I had stared at a page such as this one and seen in my own clumsy attempts to write stories just a scramble of black, or the gap between sentences—a whiteness into which we fall. And there is also a dream I have over and over again, of opening up my mouth and finding my tongue studded with broken glass, so every word is a wound.

Six weeks after Joseph had returned to school, six weeks into his failing and his ever-growing grunginess—the loss of his last hope—I went to the Museum of Science on a Saturday evening with a friend. My friend wanted to see a movie there about sharks, but because the movie was sold out, we meandered around the museum instead, finding ourselves in an exhibit about the respiratory system. Half bored, I peered my way into replicas of white lungs and lungs blackened by tar. "Cilia," a plaque read, "are small hairy outgrowths on cells. They line the lungs, the trachea, the intestinal tract. All throughout our body are cilia that act like filters, catching and then clearing away dust particles and poisons. Keeping us free from intrusive toxins, cilia are crucial to human survival."

I thought about Joseph then, and a way both to conceptualize and to work with his language problem occurred to me. Everyone's mind, I imagined, has the mental equivalent of cilia that allow for the screening out of static and the subsequent picking and choosing and shaping of ideas into sentences. Joseph, however, did not seem to have such cilia. His windpipe, lacking those little hairs, was a smooth swoop upward, spilling pennies and couches and terrors onto the page. Perhaps the problem was somehow as simple as that—not so much a damaged language capacity but a terribly untamed one that could not resist the intrusion of any subject. I recalled the sentences of his I had read, their broad beauty, their sprawling grammar that nevertheless sometimes seemed to hold seeds of meaning. And I thought of a particularly favorite passage of mine in, of all places, a neuropsychology textbook from school. This passage discussed the hypothesis that in early infancy our minds are open basins into which the whole world pours. Eventually, this theory goes, we acquire a capacity called *negative learning,* which means we become able to block out as well as let in. The specific neural ensembles responsible for negative learning have not yet been identified, but maybe, in the case of Joseph, the problem lay within those neural ensembles, those tiny microscopic screens hidden deep in gray matter.

In a way, then, Joseph was open wide and wonderful, and maybe my job was to close him, to act as some sort of screen. He didn't seem to have any screens—any cilia—of his own. If a person is born without a leg, they get a prosthetic one. What would happen, I wondered, if I acted as Joseph's prosthetic filter—a brain extension—clearing away from his sentences the verbal spasms and dust, the intrusions, that dirtied an intact meaning? Would an intact meaning then emerge? And, on a purely practical level, would I be able to help him pass his college courses? I could start to sweep. Maybe in this way, I with my broom and polishing rags, he with his ink and spit, we would learn to do a dance together; we would come to a connection.

I reached out then, rested my hand on a cell model enlarged two hundred times, a cell model covered with burgundy fuzz, tiny tentacles that waved back and forth, clearing the cluttered air.

I had an idea.

At work that Monday I looked over some of his writings. One of his sentences read, "Going back to school is a keyboard to the excellence exciting and I want to walk down the paths to the black flag beating blackboard."

Instead of looking at this sentence as crazy gibberish, I inspected it with the assumption that it was a coherent, meaningful unit, fallen victim to the breakthrough of mental dust.

Acting as Joseph's screen, I cleaned up the sentence without changing any words. The sentence now read, "Going back to school is (a keyboard to the excellence) exciting and I want to walk down the paths to the (black flag beating) blackboard."

The parentheses enclosed what I took to be the mental detritus. Further cilia scrubbing would give us: "Going back to school is exciting. I want to walk to the blackboard."

I was excited. I felt I had found something, made some sort of small discovery. A strong swath of sense really might run through many of Joseph's writings, the sediment and digressions giving them the appearance of chaos when in fact the writings were merely unedited. I tried this editing with another group of sentences, but it didn't work so easily. I had to change a lot. The sentences originally read:

> I have trouble structuring my time but I will be a gift wrapper at Jordan Marsh maybe. That's because going to Welfare is being on a treasure hunt where I eat fish and popsicles. Very confusing. Sophie got it for me. Having a job is so I don't fall into the void. It makes me feel luckyish.

Here the meaning was harder to find and, unless one knew the details of Joseph's life, reconstructing the narrative would have been difficult, if not impossible. I, however, happened to know that Sophie had been telling Joseph that he had difficulty with free time and, because of this, she was trying to get him a job at Jordan Marsh gift wrapping for the Christmas season. I suspected that Welfare, where he went to get his check each month—a building full of labyrinthine corridors and ticking clocks—somehow symbolized for Joseph a chaotic, unstructured experience. Thematically, then, the whole narrative did actually fit together. If I, acting as a bit more than a filter now, cut the welfare part and added a few left-out details and some syntactical structure, the "story" jumped into view. After I worked with it, clearing up the cluttered grammar while trying to preserve the meaning, it read:

> I have trouble structuring my time and that's why I will get a job being a gift wrapper at Jordan Marsh. My counselor Sophie will help me. I don't fall into the void if I have a job. That makes me feel luckyish.

During our session that day, I asked Joseph to write me about the things he most feared. He grabbed his pen and started his frantic scribbling, and it looked like this:

> I fear fear is fear fear fear itself fear and the invisible people in the Teddy Bear Lounge. They have all kinds of colors and I fear they are around me everywhere to go back and forth on a dream eddie talking. Where the water goes and a high cliff comes. Church is a living crab. About me and talking back at me. Everyone. They enter my mind and distract me. And I've yes always wanted to enhance myself in the present tense. They have heads and a line for a neck. Two arms and two legs. Like a geeeee!!! Charlie Brown Character!!! Their shape is distorted by . . .

And here Joseph stopped writing, started to rock. "By what, Joseph?" I asked. "Go on. Their shape is distorted by what?"

By reds and greens and white and yelllllowing the people have a girl curve feminine adventure and are GHOSSTLEY.

I had to struggle for the meaning in this one too. I had to make some assumptions about what was parenthetical and could be cut, and what was central. I had to build some verbal bridges. The work was similar not only to filtering, but also to translation when the translator does not know the native language completely, and so has to guess from context. Nevertheless, I believed that, primarily by cutting and cleaning as cilia would, I had allowed the spirit of the piece to emerge intact, and after I'd shaped it into stanzas, it read:

> I fear fear itself
> I fear invisible people
> They have all kinds of colors
> I fear they are around me, talking back at me
> They enter my mind and
> Distract me
> They have heads
> A line for a neck
> Two arms
> Two legs
> Like a Charlie Brown Character
> Their shape is distorted
> By reds and greens, whites and yellows
> The people have a girl curve

Feminine adventure and are
Ghostly

A beautiful poem, I thought, written, I thought, by
Joseph. He later titled it "Secret Illusion." The next
day I showed it to him. "Here," I said. "Here is what
you did." He took the page I'd written on, scanned it,
and his mouth dropped as he recognized his words,
cleaned and shaped. "Oh," he said. "Oh. My. Mine."
He smiled.

"Yes, yours. Another?"

"Yes."

"Your earliest memory," I said. "Write me about
your earliest memory."

And again, later on that night at my desk, I took his
scrambled prose and this time, instead of using a pen,
I typed it up. As I cut and cleaned I felt invigorated,
and close to Joseph for the first time during our treatment. The wall of babel separating him from me was
gone for a while. I could see him, hear his voice— a
boy, a bathtub, a cat calling. His pain and hopes came
clear to me. Joseph.

Pruned, his memory piece read:

I remember being washed in the sink. It's my very first
realization. It's the first memory I have of being in my
family's house, being my mother's son. She washed
me in the sink. I remember a few of the things she

said as she washed me. "Son, please beware of bad things." She said that. And that's when I was taught right from wrong. It was some kind of cleansing. She washed me in the sink every Tuesday. My mother used to give me a lot of comfort when raising me. My mother gave me a cat called Buffy. I have a picture of him and I lost it. I'm sorry I lost it.

My mom has black hair, curly. She looks like me. My mother would test me for a headache and a fever when I was young. She took very good care of me. She looked out for colds and toothaches. She always touched me. I ran in my mother's bed when I had nightmares and we would sleep together with the cat Buffy too. Dad was in the restaurant.

My mother took a heart attack a few years ago. I found her in the room, on the floor. I gave her mouth to mouth and then I called the police. I said, "My mother's on the floor." That's when my mind got worse. I got even more confused and needed structure. I started to hallucinate, the illusory things.

When I was in the sink, being washed, it was always dark. I think I felt safe in that darkness.

I don't know where she went.

Is this Joseph's real work? Can such a scrambled man take credit for a piece of prose so simplified, so smoothed? Who is *really* the author of this tale, that poem, Joseph or me? And another question: The chunks I've cut out, are they not important too, raw bits of his id tossed away like the thick fat the butcher prunes with his blades?

In shaping the tale Joseph later called "Culture of My Mother," I felt memories of my own mother returning to me (I had not seen her much in years and years, for she had left when I was fourteen), and I felt the rising rhythm in the language. Does that, then, not make me the author, possessing both the theme and the poetry of the piece? Had I been a different sort of cilia, perhaps I would have found a different sort of story in the clutter, something about mothers and trees, mothers and crabs living on a black beach.

But this is the story I heard Joseph tell me; this is the story we shaped together. And no, I think he is not any less the author because his efforts merged with mine. All stories, as Elliot Mishler, an ethnographer, claims, are "joint constructions of meaning." No author, in other words, writes a story without the pressure of an internalized culture pruning the sentences, shaping the tale.

And the tale we have here is not just about mothers; it is also about dancing. About joining. Weeks ago Joseph had trudged down a city hill, knocking on trap doors, looking for reentry. What could be more intimate than telling a tale together? How much more deeply can you enter? I lent Joseph my cells, my most private inner sieves. He felt himself falling through me. The wall of babel was gone for a time, and he did come into community—a community of me and him together. I know this is true, for often during the following days of joint creation, he touched me and murmured. He put his hand on my mouth as a lover or a mother might, and I let myself breathe into him.

And while he did finally have to drop his social psychology course, he stayed with the creative writing, passing it at the end of the semester. Sometimes I wondered what his teacher would have thought had she known my role in his writings. Would she have accused him—and me—of artistic perjury? I don't know at what point one can call a story truly one's own, where the boundaries between one mind and another's meet. I can't say that the pages you have before you here come from only me, for at every point the words—which pass from *my* axons to *my* dendrites and finally emerge in blessed sentences—are tangled in Joseph's rhythms and history, as well as in my own. Perhaps narratives are the one realm that cannot ever—despite the consumerism and capitalism in the publishing industry—be confidently claimed by any individual. I am not sure.

What I am sure of, though, is the expression on Joseph's face when I showed him the edited version of "Culture of My Mother." "You typed it up, you typed it up," he cried, as though seeing his words in print, his words graced by the daisy wheel real authors use, meant as much to him as the words themselves. "You typed it up, you typed it up," he kept chanting, and then suddenly he stopped. He held the paper up to the light as, a long time ago, his father had held up his report cards, inspecting their wondrous contents. For a second, then, he was his father and his son; he was tossed back to a past where there was hope and a wider world. And at the same time I noticed the paper I'd used was very fine—onionskin—and the light in the spare bedroom filtered through it, showing us the grains and watermarked stamp that ran like crazy currents beneath the ordered words, all that commotion threatening to well up through the streamlined sentences.

"Hello," Joseph said to the page. "Hello, my mother. My words."

Then he began to cry, softly, his face turning a tender shade of red. I, a silky piece of cilia, wanted to hold him as his mother might have, but there is only so much you can do for a patient, only so much hurt you can heal. This is what is hard about my work, knowing when to exit, knowing there are times you must take a soft touch, fingers formed into a strainer, and bring them back to your own body. Separate again.

Separate again, I watched him weep and saw there was some happiness there too. "Hello, my words," he kept saying. And with his hand he stroked and stroked the skin of the page while the page, I imagined, purred back beneath his palm, and a boy, a mother, a butter-colored cat, came alive through language.

HOLES

Every few months, when the depression becomes intolerable, Marie goes to her friend Gino's house to shoot up. The house is on top of a high hill in the inner city, and from its windows you can see silver buildings jabbing into Boston's clouds. Marie looks out those windows and then she lies next to Gino on the bed. Rubber tube, bent and rusty spoon, snow. I imagine her arms now. They are long, covered with the finest fuzz of hair, and the veins sprawl just beneath the skin. The veins rise up to the pressure of the knot, bulge blue. She shares the needle, much to my chagrin, with this man Gino, who is parchment from hepatitis, who has sores on his lips. They share the needle, exchanging not just dope but maybe something more essential, cells, molecules, the tiniest atoms, where, in each center, hexagons spin and spin with life.

She has little life, this Marie. I am so fond of her I sometimes whisper under my breath, *"My Marie."* But she is not a child and would not, probably, take well to such endearments. She wears black combat boots, tight black jeans, an old stretched sweatshirt. Most of the time she moves slowly, as if in slumber. She sleeps fifteen, sixteen hours a day, wakes just as the light loosens from the sky and drops down. When she comes to my office at the outpatient clinic, crumbs of sleep are still clustered in her eyes. "I've never been happy for more than maybe ten hours," she announces. She strokes her long arm, and I stare and stare, trying to see the needle mark, imagining a tiny hole in her skin into which I might slip, inside of which I might find the vivid parts of my Marie, yellow meadows of fat, fans of bone. Her breath.

She initially sought out treatment with me in October, my first year at the clinic, because, as she put it, "I cannot take being depressed anymore."

Depression, I thought to myself then. It's a psychiatric disorder suffered by one in ten Americans and, despite the severe pain an all-out bout can inflict— lack of appetite, dwindled sex drive, crying jags that last for hours—it's still remarkably banal, as common as the common cold. At its best, I viewed depression as a bronchitis of the brain, undeniably difficult but not nearly as exciting as the holy lights and purple pumpkins conjured up by my psychotic patients. I didn't know then—although I soon would—how even the plainest ills can yield the most exotic questions. I was not aware of how my work with Marie would turn me back toward memories of myself—a skinny girl in an empty house, a blank, flat world where all sounds ceased—and then turn me outward, to the very rim of the sky, where we humans hope to see the red eye of Mars, the open mouth of the moon, as a part of some god's face.

But I'm ahead of myself. She didn't come to me for reasons that had to do with God. At five feet seven inches tall, she weighed in at just over a hundred pounds. Her eyes seemed to slouch in their sockets and her skin had the damp, whitish look of larvae.

"For how long has it been like this?" I asked.

"Forever," she said. "Just about for—" She stopped. "I don't know how—" Stopped again. And stared out the window, stared at the ceiling, such long pauses between her utterances I wondered if she'd forgotten them, all words disappearing into the mud of her mind.

"Forever?" I prompted. "You said forever?"

She turned her gaze back to me. "It's always been a fucking battle," Marie said. "Sometimes a little bit easier, sometimes a little bit harder. And every once in a while, presto." She snapped her fingers. Her nails were painted a cracked peach, and one of them was pierced with a tiny gold hoop. "For a few hours or days it completely disappears. I'm fine. It's great. But the depression always comes back."

She went on, in her slow, stop-and-start voice, to explain how she'd never held down a job because of her grief, how she'd been on every antidepressant medication then available (this was before Prozac) and had improved on none. Her condition caused her days of paralysis, and, as a result, she lived with her two children in a barely furnished apartment in one of the city's housing projects. "If I could feel better for anything more than a couple of split seconds," she said to me that first session, "then maybe I'd have the energy to get off welfare and stay with a job long enough to make real money."

I had a lot of optimism when I first started with Marie. If one in ten Americans suffer at some point in their lives from this kind of major depression, well over 90 percent of them recover. Why shouldn't she? Despite the seriousness of the disorder, it's considered highly treatable, either through medication, which had so far failed her, or through the standard fare of talk therapy, which we would now try. And talk therapy—the type I practice at the outpatient clinic—

almost always begins at the beginning, by inquiring into the patient's past. Somewhere in my mind I thought her seemingly inexorable depression stemmed from childhood wounds. This theory, originally set forth by Freud, sets psychological healing as analogous to a surgical procedure. The past is pus. The patient talks about it, her tongue like the surgeon's scalpel that scrapes the wound clean. Dabbed and dried, the poison now drained, the abrasion can begin to heal. What a simplistic approach this now seems to me, what a borrowed metaphor—science, surgery, superimposed upon a process where no one has been able to locate an actual disease. You cannot, after all, see depression. There are no really reliable tests to measure for it. A woman can give a cup of urine and from its fauna the doctor can determine the life of the liver, or the hormones that begin a baby. A man can give a vial of blood and in its cells the phlebotomist can detect the specific virus that will kill him. Scrape anywhere on the body, though—measure a hair, probe a pore—and nowhere will you touch or view the deep grief that is depression. This might suggest to us that depression does not exist in the medical sense, and that a medical model for its treatment might be poorly conceived. Never mind that, though. It's how I was trained. I began with what I knew how to do.

· · ·

I began by extracting details from her, the elements of her history, and while now I am not so sure how relevant these elements are to the specifics of her suffering, I will set them forth here because they are a part of my Marie, the plot from which she springs.

In the beginning, then, we had a girl who wanted to be a nurse. One day her mother took her to St. Margaret's clinic to have a splinter removed—her father usually did these kinds of things, but he was away somewhere—and then she saw the nurses in their starched long skirts, the fresh red crosses stitched to their breast pockets. It must have been the contrasts that enchanted her, the hemoglobin richness set against the cleanest winter, red burning through bleach. She recalled a nurse soaking her swollen finger in a bowl of salt water, and then tweezers entering her sore skin, withdrawing the wood, sending her to the peak of pain, and then the lovely coolness of crushed ice.

This was comfort, something her own home didn't have much of. The plaster walls there were full of holes. Her father was a muscular man who worked as a day laborer, making one dollar and fifty-two cents an hour. His comfort was vodka, his release a rage that could send Marie or one of her sisters slamming against a wall. Her mother's comfort was food and fatness. Nights, her father would sit in the den, shot glass in his hand, and her mother, blank and apathetic, would sit in the kitchen in an old housecoat, plates of macaroni before her. During the early days of therapy, Marie told me a story about her mother that has since been with me. It was right after a bath, her mother—dewlapped and pockmarked—stepping from the tub and Marie walking in by accident. The enormous woman rose from the steam, set one bare leg on the floor. It was the leg that haunted Marie, the leg that still today sends shudders through her. Its ankle was bloated and marred with a mysterious excrescence, not a pimple, not a wart or a bunion. Something considerably larger, something red-purplish and hook-shaped. Marie was five, maybe six. She crept forward to see. Above her, this mountain of a mother dried herself off, terry cloth slapping on swinging flesh. Marie crawled toward the ankle, reached her hand forward. The growth rose up, spiked all over with stiff black hairs. Was it a cactus coming from inside the body, a reptilian tail like the kind she'd seen on lizards at school? Marie uncurled her finger—everything in her recoiling and reaching at the same time—and pressed the protuberance, felt how hard it was, how scaly, and then she realized it was some kind of claw growing from her mother's flesh.

"Like she was a witch," Marie said to me during the first few months of therapy. "Like I lived in a place that was cursed." Soon after that incident she started to play nurse with her dolls and her sisters. From their flesh she extracted imaginary splinters, waved the wand of her hand and caused chasms to close. For months and months after school, in that house where rage and sadness simmered, Marie ripped up old sheets, made long bandages she would lovingly wrap around limbs. Such soothing.

"There was no soothing where you grew up," I said to her. "Your father abused you, your mother frightened you. Tell me more."

I asked her to tell me more because I was betting on a cycle of reconnecting and remembering, the tongue exorcising the trauma. Because I thought if a patient could talk about the trauma, bring it to consciousness, then she could eject it. Once ejected, such a patient would be free to refashion the trauma, to reclaim it in new form, much the way a doctor gently lifts the heart from its socket, cleans the wheezing arteries, and then sets it back in its bed of muscle.

But this is not exactly what happened with Marie. Talking about her past—that combination of catharsis and insight—did little to relieve her pain. Week after week she came dragging her depression to treatment. She did occasionally have "good days," but, as she had told me at the very outset, these good days had occurred throughout her life, brief periods of time when the pain would pull back and Marie would experience the world on a surprisingly different slant. These slants didn't seem to be happening any more frequently since we'd begun working together, nor did they seem at all connected to any insight or conversation or catharsis. They were random remissions that occurred as she stared into the bowl on the mantel in a friend's home, or as she walked on the pavement and looked down at the concrete cracks webbed within. These remissions zinged out of nowhere, and because she could not count on them, nor will them, they remained in her mind as treasures she felt entirely out of control of and entirely grateful to, a potent and ambivalent combination.

"Sometimes," Marie said to me, "it happens when I'm in the shower. Or when I step out of the shower and the water begins to dry on my skin. There's a . . . a lifting."

And I, too, lifted, leaned forward in my seat. I thought of fevers lifting, dew lifting and leaving the grass a cleaner green. In her words I heard a surge of hope, and because hope is what we all finally want, what we are all entranced by, I held to it.

"Explain," I said.

And so she did. Over a series of meetings, she explained these moments to me. "I was once walking by a chapel," she said, "and the bells began to gong. It was like each gong cracked into the depression. Then everything felt different." And as she described these moments to me, her own voice sounded different, the flat plodding taking on rise, rhythm. "So I went right inside and an excitement came over me, so *great*. The saints seemed to be singing." And then she went on to tell me how she stood there, transfixed, how the dusk in the stained glass was gentle and the candles wept a clean white wax, a warmth she wanted to touch. "I felt unbelievably alive," Marie said.

"If only you could keep that aliveness," I murmured, and I was thinking then of moments in my own life when the world had presented itself to me all shucked and gleaming. How once, in England, I had gone to a dilapidated cathedral, where images of angels were etched in the walls, and found, in the tiny cracks between the graying stones, beautiful swatches of emerald moss and pearl-like pebbles. How our own bodies are like that too, opalescent paths tucked between skins we can't see. Is that a condition of being human, to lose light, to lose sight of the special angles? Was Marie just an exaggeration of us all, all of us walking a plain path, privy every once in a while to a vision more essential, a vision we can't keep? How often you hear people complain that daily life is a drag, that it is better not to fall in love than to endure the pain of falling out, back into banality.

"And when these moments go away," Marie said, "I want them back and then I wish they never came because things feel even harder afterward."

Sometimes, Marie told me, these moments would stretch out into a couple of days, or if she were really on a roll, maybe even into a few weeks. During these hours she would scrub her house, pay stacks of bills, return the messages cluttering up her phone machine. She would rise very early, at five A.M., and stay up past midnight. "I can't let myself sleep too much," Marie said, "because I have energy and it's my one chance to get things done." She knew, in other words, that once the depression returned, these ordinary tasks would become overwhelming, how the sound of a dial tone would burn in her ear, how fatigue would loosen her limbs, so even holding a sponge—that meringue from the sea, all airiness and ripples—would feel too hard, too heavy.

"I'm living with a remote control inside my head. It doesn't feel like I have a choice. A person I can't see presses the up button and I feel better. I'm washing my dishes, doing all this stuff. I'm singing. And then right in the middle of the tune this invisible person presses the down button. And then I can't even open my mouth."

Four months into treatment, a remission came. Marie strode into my office one afternoon with lively eyes. "Yup," she said to me, sitting down, "I'm in a good mood, an excellent mood. Since last Thursday. Six days now." She leaned forward, counting off on her fingers and dropping her voice. "Six days and it's awesome."

I wondered about mania, the flip side of depression, where the mood zooms up too high and happiness turns crazy. But none of the signs were there. Her speech was normal, her thinking intact. "I'm eating OK, I'm sleeping OK once I actually get to bed. I mean I'm staying up late so I can do all the stuff I've been putting off, but I'm out soon as I hit the pillow. I'm just enjoying myself," she added.

I nodded, sat back in my seat. I was seeing her for the first time without the jammed grief. I noticed the wet whiteness of her teeth. I noticed—had it always been there?—the soft green snake of a vein in her temple. If I watched the vein for long enough I thought I could see the splutter of her pulse. And then relief went through me. Every helper wants to ease some suffering. The greater the suffering, the greater the sense of responsibility. For a moment I didn't have that pressure. And I could for the first time see Marie as the woman she might be able to be.

"In the welfare office today I saw an advertisement," she said. "Job training. I actually signed up."

And it was true. This woman, usually so paralyzed, now went ahead into vocational training. For the next few weeks, while her children were in school, Marie hustled off every day to a building in Chelsea, where, with fourteen other welfare mothers, she learned to mend computer hardware. She learned, in her lightness and energy, how to pry loose the faulty silicon chips, clip the veins of wire braided over the bus, reknot so a fresh supply of energy flowed in. I saw her as a doctor in some strange ritual of mending, she probing for viruses among infected hardware, the profound gratification of finding the ill chip and plucking it, like an abscessed tooth, from the motherboard's jaw.

I suppose I knew this interlude would be just that. She had told me about her pattern. So I should have been prepared when, one morning, three weeks into her fine mood, I got a call from an emergency-room physician telling me that Marie had overdosed. Could I please give him some background information?

I don't really remember what he asked me for, or what information I gave. Instead I was going back over the past few weeks, searching for signs. Did I see sweat on her forehead yesterday, something sad in her eyes? Had she been starting to speak and move more slowly again? I looked among my memories, my notes. I am in a line of work, after all, that venerates origins, that grasps for reasons and roots: "If this happened, it was because of this. If you stare into an aqua bowl and find yourself smiling, it is because you see the color of the ocean, remember primitive blue and blood, how for nine months you rode close to your mother's walls, her waves."

Maybe, then, something in those machines reminded her of her early home. Maybe their ordered loveliness contrasted too sharply with the chaos of her history. Maybe in touching the thick and beautiful wires of the motherboard, she remembered, by contrast, the cold spikes in her mother's skin, and a secret grief reopened. Or maybe not. "No reason I can see," she muttered to me later, through cracked lips, as she lay in her hospital bed. I didn't want there to be no reason, just a sudden, senseless resurgence. It went against everything I had learned, everything I needed to believe—that psychological pain occurs for a solid reason and rests, therefore, on some solid sense.

But this isn't how she described it, Marie. That evening, in the emergency room, she told me in a slow flat voice how she had woken up in the morning and felt the gritty light of the sun scorch her eyes. There had been no fight, no nightmare, no put-down in school. She had, simply, gone to sleep in one state and woken up in another. "No dream?" I said, straining forward on the hospital bed. "No memory of something bad?"

Marie shook her head. She had just woken up that morning and felt the dread of that depression back on her. She had tried to get out of bed and found she could barely move. The idea of facing what just yesterday she had loved appalled her. The wires would look ugly, rotting tendons on greased machines. The gas plasma screens would reek, glow a fetid green. She couldn't go. She just couldn't go. Her heart hammered and every second squeezed inside. Morning passed into noon, noon into dusk. The dusk was dirty and her face in the mirror looked streaked with soot. She knew the few weeks of energy, the few weeks where she had had the capacity again to experience love, were gone. When her children came home she would not recognize them, their teeth like tombstones, the holes in their noses too wide. She rushed out of the house.

She told me all of this slowly as I sat on the edge of the hospital bed. She looked up at the ceiling, her voice as bleak as a British moor. Some of the color and drama I add, the way someone salts her food, wishing away the bland paleness of her plate.

And so she had rushed out of the house and up the hill to Gino's. The needle in her skin felt good, felt something. She didn't put it in her arm but in her chest, in the ravine between the breasts, shooting directly into the large thick vein over the heart. In an instant a white and cottony relief enveloped her, and, before she dropped into an unconscious dream, she envisioned her body as the inside of a machine, all the parts gleaming, the silicon slab of her heart recharged, relieved.

An accidental overdose, meant for relief, not death. The emergency-room doctor told me she had railed against the Naloxone they'd injected into her to block the opiate's action. After she was medically cleared, the plan was to transfer her to the hospital's psychiatric floor until she was stable again. When I had gone to see her that evening, I had looked into her face, barely distinguishable from the paleness of the pillow, and I didn't know what to do, how to explain this strange cycle of suffering and redemption either to her or to myself.

She was on the psychiatric unit for two days. I went to visit her there once. The charge nurse told me Marie refused to come out of her room except to spend hours in a toilet stall, that she wept constantly and absolutely would not attend groups.

I was actually happy to hear about Marie's refusal to go to groups. It spoke of some spark of anger, some spot still scarlet within her. When I heard that, I got yet another glimpse of Marie, this time not joyful, nor flattened by grief, but lit red in her rage. Imagine, to love over and over again, and then to lose the love. Imagine fighting your way through days, sudden spurts of light, and then drought. Depression is a death within, a knowledge—terrifying—that you cannot resurrect yourself. Depression is loss of the vision that lets leaves breathe and fall, that lets the air smell of seed and soil. And there must be rage, yes I think there is rage toward such a severing, such a ragged-deep rupture with the world.

She was in her room, sitting on a chair pulled up to the window. Below her, patients wandered around a fenced lawn.

I drew up a chair and sat beside Marie. For a long time we said nothing. I searched her profile, as though in its angles I might find clues about what to do next.

"I don't understand it," she finally said. "But as long as I go on this way, I'll never accomplish anything."

"School," I said. "Like school."

"Fuck that," she spit. "My children. *The air.*"

"The air?"

"It's like I forget how to breathe." She hunched over herself. "And when that happens I'll do anything to get my breath back. Heroin helps."

"What makes you want to keep on breathing? I mean, why do you keep swimming to shore, after all these years? Do you ever think of just letting yourself drown?"

"Yes, I do," Marie said.

"What stops you?" My voice cracked. It's frightening to speak of death directly, especially death as a choice. Even though all the writings on suicide say talking about it will never put such an idea, or worse, such an impulse, into someone's head, I've always been hesitant anyway. Maybe because to speak of something is to radically reveal it, and suddenly Marie and I were swimming, or drowning, in some new space.

"I don't know," Marie said. She slowly shook her head. "Every time it gets this bad, I think, 'Marie, you know it'll get better. You have your good days. Your great days, even.' I remember my moments, because whenever I have them, I think, 'This time it'll last. This is so fucking good.' And so I hang on. And on."

She stopped. It was evening now, and outside a searchlight angled across the city sky. Where did that light come from—I saw it almost every night, from my car window, my bedroom window, my office window, arcing rhythmically across the smoggy air, then shriveling back to its unseen beginnings, only to sprout again a moment later. Even as a little girl (I've lived in this city all of my life) I'd seen that light, and the woman who took care of me after my parents had left for good used to make up stories about its source, how it came from a magician's tower, how it was a warlock's flashlight and he used it to illuminate the woods he walked through. Then I was no longer in the city, or in a home where there were no parents, but way out on the edge of things, on the border where magic happens and enormous, impossible flowers struggle up through blue soil. These are the moments we make or are given to celebrate ourselves, the moments that redeem our regular or tired lives.

We wait for them, still breathing.

These days, the managed-care health system demands that a patient be discharged as soon as the imminent danger has passed. There's no extra time for staff to do aftercare planning or simply soothe a tired mind. "Are you feeling suicidal or self-destructive today?" the hospital staff must ask. And if the patient answers no, fiscal concerns demand discharge, despite the fact that, like a searchlight, such a suicidal urge may come again tomorrow, sweeping across the psyche's sky.

So it was that Marie, with barely enough energy to talk, was released from the psychiatric unit within forty-eight hours. She was no longer considered "a danger to self or others." She was given two subway tokens and told to make her way back home. Because home was far from the hospital, though, the subway tokens covered only half her trip. Without money, then, and still sluggish, she found herself lost in the center of a busy downtown and was forced to spend the night in a homeless shelter, on a cot amid a row of cots and rumpled women whose breath smelled of beer and ash. By the time she made it to her appointment with me the following day, her face and hair were damp with oil and her lips were chapped, the fissures bleeding lightly.

Seeing her, I panicked. I wanted lotions and soaps, cups of steeped tea I could feed her. I wanted—an urge so strong it surprised me—to make her a meal, that wish for eggs I could crack against a steaming skillet, the gentleness of yolks.

"Marie, Marie," I said softly.

She cried in my office that day, head in cupped hands, body bent. "I don't know," she kept repeating.

"We'll figure this out," I said, but I wasn't very sure.

I had learned other methods of working with depression, and over the next few months of therapy we would try them out. Insight, obviously, had been a failure. Something else had to work. My panic came from real failure, but more so from being overwhelmed. Who wants to witness hurting in another? Who wants to stand by and watch blood? Better to bandage it up. Now I think I know—although I didn't then—that sometimes all we can do is align ourselves with the wound, respect its oozings and witness its crimson colors. Sometimes all we can do is keep company with the person who hurts. I did not know then that this in and of itself just might constitute help.

Help would be to make better, to relieve. So we tried something called cognitive therapy, the main point of which was to get Marie to alter her attitude toward pain. This kind of treatment springs from work with patients who have had chronic physical illnesses. The theory goes that if patients can learn not to react with anxiety or tension when they have a bad sensation, if they can learn to relax and accept the pain, they will lessen the grip the suffering has over their skin. In other words, pain does not exist apart from perception, and if a patient can change her perception of pain, then she has, in effect, changed the pain itself.

Marie and I worked on tweaking her perception of pain. Was it really as bad as she thought it was? How many hours a day was she actually depressed, and could she log those hours in a book? By logging them, did she begin to notice that things weren't quite as terrible as she assumed? Could she practice saying to herself, "This hurts but it won't kill me? This is only a feeling, not a fact?"

Marie's response to this treatment after some weeks: "Yes, it's only a feeling but it still does hurt. No, I'm not overestimating my depression and the number of hours a day I feel it. What you want," she said to me, "is for me to be less depressed about being depressed." She shrugged. "I can't accept that."

We tried looking at depression from a feminist perspective and engendering some sort of political anger on her part. No go. We tried a purely behavioral approach—Marie forcing herself up out of bed, calling three friends a day, showering regularly. No go. One night during this time I was at a friend's house and I picked up the remote control for the television. I pressed 1, 2, 3. I pressed > for volume up and < for volume down. I pictured Marie miles and miles away, her mind twitching and swirling as I held the electrical box, a yellow slice of sun edging over the rim of her brain, a saint placing some cool moss on her forehead. Emerald. Transfixed by dusk. A door opening, sand and water. *Walk there, Marie,* I thought. *Can you wait for one of those moments?*

This all happened at the particular moment in medication history when Prozac was emerging. Marie had been tried on the entire range of antidepressant medication over the years of her illness, but none had done the trick. Now we were just beginning to learn about this new kind of medication that had had some grand successes. *Just maybe,* we thought, *it will work.* Marie was hopeful. I knew something about how Prozac had been made, how, unlike other psychiatric medications, it had been designed to cut a clear path to the problem in the brain, acting on a certain specific neurotransmitter. Whereas the older types of antidepressants were clumsy in their actions, tweaking all sorts of unnecessary synapses in their stumbling journey to the particular sore spot and causing, therefore, a whole range of unpleasant side effects, Prozac was like a supremely coordinated athlete, a hurdle jumper who cleared every fence and arrived at the finish line with sure, smooth strides. Whether or not this image is precisely true, I cannot say. I would suspect not. But this is the myth that was already growing around the capsule, the image that at least in part propelled a national fervor. When you swallowed Prozac you were swallowing not just a pill, but a technical triumph, a bionic piece of biology.

A week after her discharge from the hospital, Marie saw the outpatient clinic's psychiatrist, who prescribed her Prozac. Twice a day now, once in the morning and once in the evening, she ingested her pills. I pictured her standing by the kitchen window, a glass of water, the amber bottle. It would take several weeks to work. Now we had to wait.

Once I had read a series of accounts about some amazing and sickening brain operations. I can't recall all the places I found these accounts, because this was a long time ago, well before I knew Marie. But the images from these surgical descriptions returned to me just at this point in our treatment.

I recalled reading of a man lying on an operating table. Surgeons hovered around him. In the patient's head was a hole caused by a cancer that had eaten through the patient's scalp, revealing the brain, gray and pink, surrounded by cerebral fluid that now and then burbled over and dripped down the man's stripped scalp. When that happened, one of the attending nurses would dab at the wound with a sterile cloth, wiping away the wetness. The doctors, in the meantime, cut away at the cancerous hunk of head and went about inserting a metal plate. The patient would live, but with great gaps in his mind, memories of flowers and words snipped from his skull and tossed. Was it worth the price? I had wondered. Would it have been better to simply have let the sick man die? To what lengths will we travel in order to "heal," and why does "healing" always imply a triumph over illness as opposed to an acknowledgment of it?

Yes, it was at this point that I remembered reading about these operations and the questions they had then, and now, brought forth in me. Because twice a day Marie swallowed her pills and nothing happened, even after weeks and weeks. It's not that I then thought I should advocate suicide. It was more that I, like those gloved surgeons, could not accept the naked pain, could not stop trying to cut and clean, to remove the stone of suffering that sometimes sits in the center of our lives. Modern medicine, of which psychiatry and psychology are a part, is, as the critic David Morris writes, "fundamentally anti-tragic in [its] vision, simply cannot go on gripped by a vision of permanent defeat."

And yet here we were, Marie and I, defeated. Ten, eleven, twelve weeks went by and the Prozac did not, as they say, kick in. I went home then, and lay on my bed. Marie went home and lay on hers. Although I was not the depressed one here, I felt tired, felt I had come to the very edge of my efforts. I closed my eyes and dropped down. At the bottom of the hole, past the push of scalpels, lies that unalterable stone of suffering. I could see the stone now, in half-sleep—deep blue, raw coral. Maybe the job was not to remove it, but to more clearly delineate its meaning in her life. Could I call myself a modern "helper," a "doctor," of some sort, if I gave in to pain's nervy power instead of trying to triumph over it? There is little place in the halls of the contemporary clinic for this kind of thinking. It's what I was thinking. I saw again the hole in that man's head, the way the fluid had edged over, how the nurses wiped it up. Maybe, instead, they should have gathered the fluid in cupped hands, lifted it to their lips, tasting within it a briny memory of how we are born howling, a salty nerve cell, a whole network of nerves whose purpose is pleasure but also pain, without which we are not who we are—human.

And so I began, slowly, in knowing Marie, to think about staying in suffering instead of always trying to climb out of it. Do not mistake me. I don't mean I learned to embrace pain, whose boiling body frightens me as it scalds the skin of its victims, nor, in the parlance of New Age–speak, to accept pain, for acceptance is far too sweet a word, and I doubt very many people loosen their limbs and lie pliantly in the lap of hurting. I mean I learned, quite simply—in these technical times, when the hope for new remedies is daily dangled before our eyes—to acknowledge pain, to sit still in its mysterious presence and feel helpless.

I gave up. No more interventions. No more pithy observations or attempts at radical reconstructions. Our sessions took, in the following days, a bit of a different turn. "Perhaps," I said to Marie after the psychiatrist had discontinued the Prozac, "you won't overcome your depression. Perhaps you'll have to . . . have to learn to live with it."

Those words jammed up my gullet. I felt as though I were betraying something, and I recalled again the words of David Morris:

> Our culture teaches us to confront pain with silence and denial. Americans today probably belong to the first generation on earth that looks at a pain-free life as something like a constitutional right. Pain is a scandal.

"Well, what would that mean?" Marie said.

I didn't know. We sat thinking about it, and it felt as if there were a string stretched between us. The string was not a lifeline I had thrown her, but the raw tendon that connects people at the moment both become willing to enter a wound—an intimacy arises as they go down, past pulses and neurons and bones buffed smooth. And in that unknown place they wait, the two together, holding hands.

The seasons passed. By Easter there was a clearer focus to our endeavors. We ceased discussing ways of beating the depression and instead explored how she might know it as an essential part of her. Jung said that the point of therapy is to become what you fundamentally are, the figures hunched within, fully formed from the moment of birth, or before birth, from the moment sperm meets seed and cells take shape. I can't in any way claim Marie was happy about this new way we walked, but something felt right in our strides, as if we'd reached a rhythm. Still, I wondered, what kind of rhythm was it? What kind of plot did we have here? Marie certainly still spent days bleary with pain, and if there's any epiphany in this tale, any kind of crescendo, it comes at least as much from my need to shape a narration of progress—what after all, is therapy, if not a story of progress?—as it does from her experience.

But maybe, just maybe, we should cease thinking of therapy as a story moving forward. Such a story could be harmful to people who are bound to feel like failures in a milieu where the expectation of improvement is so clearly etched. Perhaps the therapist's job is not to help grow but to help shed, chipping away at the marbled mind until the original nubs and spurs emerge. Instead of thinking in terms of development, maybe we should be thinking in terms of sloughing, making the padded self thinner and thinner until a true skeleton juts out. And who says, who ever said, we would want to celebrate a skeleton? Who said it would redeem us? For Marie was still slow in her speech, in her gait. Nevertheless, I thought I saw some kind of attentiveness in the way she leaned forward in her seat, as though our discussions now touched the pulse point of how she lived. She no longer "complied" with my interventions, or dutifully laid bare the facts of her early life, but went with me into marrow. Or perhaps I should say I went with her, for I was the one now learning about pain. She was the one now living in it.

And when we looked out the window of my office, we saw rain silvered in a streetlight. We saw the frailest of halos. Black umbrellas were as sleek as the coats of seals. I began to notice small things as therapy continued, and sometimes my sight felt so clear objects were transformed, so the pale fuzz on my lover's nape deepened to gold, a field of soft wheat in the summer. I wondered then if I was taking on some of Marie's heightened moments, some of her occasional spasms of joy. I wondered if, in traveling with me into the wound, she had, inadvertently, shown me a place of clear color and exceptional angles.

During those sessions we discussed the ways throughout history that people have tried to make sense of their suffering, old myths about Navajo bones beginning to rise, men coming back as birds.

"Well, what about those saints?" Marie said. "Like Sebastian. What do you think he actually saw as he was nailed?"

"Oh, I don't know. Angels, maybe? Sunlight?"

Marie smiled then. "Computers," she said. "Those little silicon chips and how they all go together when you're having a good day."

"Do you ever wonder," I asked, "whether your depression is what actually gives you such good moments? I mean, maybe one of the things your pain does is to bring you a kind of sharpness of vision."

"Maybe," Marie said.

I nodded.

"But big whoop-de-do." She glared at me. "That's a fucking high price to pay for a few good times."

"Those times have kept you alive, though, haven't they?" I was recalling what she had said to me in the hospital, about why she had not chosen suicide.

Marie paused. "It's pretty incredible," she said, "that I'm such a fool, that I stick around day after day, month after month, just waiting for one of my little breaks of sunshine."

There was anger in her voice, rage, even, and the rage told me this: that Marie was a woman of great faith, and her faith was formed by a brief succession of seconds that never lasted. She lived out months, years of pain on the hope of again experiencing those brief remissions, those slivers of time when the world went shucked, went gleaming. And while we usually celebrate faith, I saw just then how cruel it can be, if I were to push it, how even pathological are those tough tethers of pleasure that keep us anchored to an earth we can little enjoy.

I looked closely at Marie then. My Marie. We had found no answers at all, but we had come to questions we could ask together. And the questions seemed so dignified—*what does my wound mean?* And her wondering and walking in the rawest places seemed so brave that, watching her, I came to know all it might mean to be human.

And maybe what it means to be human is this. Maybe it means looking down, down, until you see a naked ankle out of which grows a mound of purplish flesh, a lump beating with a horrible heart you yearn to touch anyway. Maybe it means such spreads of silence new sounds are born, and you hear the weeping of fish, the crying inside the ocean. As a child, after my parents had left, I moved into a house where there was an old tree with a gaping trunk hole in the backyard. During the day I went outside and stared into the trunk, stared into that mossy hole, as surgeons stare into the scalp of some moribund man. Being human, maybe, means looking into holes, propelled by a belief that something lives at the end of their length. So I peered through there, straight into the torso of that tree, even though the odor of the dead wood and the shining flecks of termites made me queasy, and I wanted to turn away. I didn't. Instead, a bit like my Marie, I kept on, almost compulsively, staring past the moss, the scurrying insects, through to the very heart of the rot, where, deep inside the oak, stagnant water gathered. Where worms lay coiled in a smelly silt. Where tree toads lived, whole flocks of toads who blinked back at me, twelve gold gazes, twelve croaking throats. Yes. Twelve gold gazes, a sweep of something lovely that kept me, us—fools?—hooked and hoping, still.

A GREAT WIND

There's a garden in back of the ward. In it grow tiny pink roses, crocuses, and each summer rich red tomatoes and silvery stalks of corn. In the year and a half that I've now worked here, I've come to use the garden to measure the men's progress. I have my own small system worked out, a system set apart, of course, from the graphs and codes mental-health professionals usually use to chart the undulations of illness. If I see a man lean over and gently touch a thorn, I think the flat gloss of his psychosis may be waning, the world reemerging for him in all its angles and prongs. If I observe a patient compulsively fingering a cluster of berries swimming in the air like tiny bubbles of blood, I get a bad feeling, worry about the violence that sometimes accompanies craziness. I've decided smelling is a good sign, tasting yet a better one; touching can go either way. The mention of colors delights me, as when Moxi announced the other day how he loved the "greening grass." And then there are the men who seem not to see any color at all, who, when brought out to the garden, wend their way through, stumbling and clumsy, and I think that indicates a poor prognosis.

Of all the patients on the ward, the catatonics are the most immune to the garden. Thus, although some textbooks claim catatonia—very rare these days, anyway—is a less severe form of schizophrenia than other subsets of the disease, I would have to disagree. Sometimes in group I've asked my men to draw the verdant growth out back, and the catatonics have failed terribly at this task. We once had a catatonic who stayed on the ward for only two months. His name was Harold, and when presented with a fan of vibrant Crayolas with which to capture the bloom and duff of bushes, of flowers, he chose only white. The paper was white, the wax Crayola was white, and the finished project was invisible except for the occasional sad shimmer of some mysterious curlicues. Four days after that, Harold, in a stupor, choked on his own vomit and had to be transferred to a medical hospital.

Catatonia is haunting precisely because it flirts so closely with images of death. Tomography scans of catatonic schizophrenics' brains show major damage, the nerve cells thinned and the areas that are supposed to be rich in nourishing glial cells starved bare and brown. Case studies of the catatonics who actually house these brains describe patients pretzled in the same position for years and years, their bodies spasmed and stiff in a dark, fetid-smelling room, while beyond the closed curtains the earth pumps up flowers and then sucks the stems back to die. Other times, catatonia is less dramatic. Even someone who walks and talks can show signs of the disorder, in the slowed speech or senseless repetitive movements, in a dullness of the eyes. Simply put, the catatonic is someone unresponsive to the environment, and because unresponsiveness occurs on a continuum, so, too, may its consequences. Neuropsychologists have discovered that one of these consequences is sometimes a condition called *agraphesthesia,* which means that if you trace a number or a letter on the catatonic's skin, he may not be able to sense it's a plump 8 or a stern *A* or the tiny teacup of a *u.* His skin is not a sponge, as all good skin should be, absorbing the world, reading within its pores the curves and textures that shape the stories of our lives.

Of the schizophrenics I've worked with, Oscar DiBenedetto is the one who, in his very stillness, has moved me the most. He's the forty-one-year-old mustached man, the one who loves albinos and sketches empty skulls. He is heaped with fat. No matter what the weather, Oscar often insists upon wearing a wool hat, wool mittens, and a scarf knotted around his neck. Black stiff hairs spike from his nose and ears, and in the heat of the summer his pitted face shines with sweat that drips from his chin and darkens his woolen wraps. Oscar has been diagnosed with, among other things, schizophrenia, catatonic type. This means that at his worst he's dumb and frozen for days, sitting in a chair or on his bed and staring out at the world, compulsively clicking his tongue and unresponsive to anything around him. At his best, Oscar is stuporous and slow, and in between he's frantic from some of the most terrifying hallucinations I've ever heard of.

Because Oscar moves so little, and when he does it's mostly to eat, his weight's a big problem on the ward. So is his smell. Staff despair of ever getting Oscar to run his own bath or shed some pounds. In the year and a half I've worked on the ward, Oscar has already broken five chairs just by sitting in them, and no one can leave leftovers in the refrigerator because, as long as he's not locked in one of his dazes, Oscar will devour them. At two A.M., staff have sometimes caught him standing by the light of the open refrigerator, emptying dishes with his hands. Once I did an overnight and discovered Oscar thus—what an eerie sight, this enormously fat man standing in shadows, hooded and earmuffed, sauteed livers hanging from his lips.

"Oscar, what are you doing?" I asked.

He turned around, shrugged. "Snacking."

"At three in the morning?"

Oscar looked at the kitchen clock, a glowing disc with a second hand sailing in silent circles. "It's not three," he finally said. "It's a quarter to three."

"Well, why don't you get on back to bed?" I suggested.

"Yeah, bed," Oscar said, "my bed," and then he shuffled off, leaving the refrigerator wide open and the counter full of food. I went forward to see the midnight feast, as if perhaps in its crumbs and colors I might find some clue about this man, the heat and urges behind his glassed-in flatness. I didn't get much. On the counter lay a plate of congealed gravy, the pit from some fruit, and spareribs cleansed of any meat, the bones sucked smooth as sleep.

Sleep isn't really what catatonics drop into when they become completely mute, but rather a daze born of fear. Experiments have revealed that human beings aren't the only animals who show catatonia, or what is also sometimes called the immobility response. Flip an alligator on its back and its entire body becomes pliant. Before slaughter, rabbits dangled upside down by their back feet go into a stupor, as though they know their imminent deaths, can even see how later they will hang on hooks in the butcher's frosted vault. The immobility response is the last adaptive mechanism in a series of stages animals go through when they sense their demise. First there is running, squawking, hiding, and then, at last, this stillness, so complete the brain shuts down except for a tiny red flicker deep in its hemispheres. This flicker keeps the heart beating and the blood from going cold, but the nerves that web the body dream. There's no pain as the teeth sink in or the noose does its choking work. In one experiment, frogs were released in the presence of a ferret. The ferret poked out its pointy head and chewed off one frog's legs, another's eye. The frogs froze. They appeared to feel nothing. This comforts me and also strangely saddens me. I know there are limits to the horrors of the world. I also know our bodies sometimes leave us before we have left them.

In the natural world of woods and fields, dangers can be charted. Hawks and vultures swarm a stone-blue sky. Wasps carry a paralyzing agent within their glands, which they slowly inject into a helpless cicada while the wasp's newly hatched larvae eat the cicada alive. But in Oscar's world, the dangers are harder to grasp. We know only what he manages to tell us, or what sketchy records indicate.

His records report he's the only child of Victoria and Cecil DiBenedetto, whose marriage ended in divorce when Oscar was fifteen. Cecil, apparently, had been molesting Oscar nightly, and when the mother discovered this, she threw her husband out. Four months into divorce proceedings, while Victoria was cleaning out Cecil's dresser, she came across black scrolls of film that showed her son's body nude and angled, stretched and probed. Pornography, hours and hours of it, her son's broadening chest and hairs crammed into this camera. Later it turned out that the father was part of a huge child-pornography ring in Revere. Oscar has never spoken of his father's abuses, or of those strange filming sessions he underwent with twenty-five other boys. He has never spoken directly of rape, the clicking camera, and lights searing his skin. He has never mentioned the frills he was forced to wear, the way the zippers must have felt, or the oiled look of a crop. If you ask him about that time in buried basements, he starts to chatter and rock, or he says something strangely, poetically apt, as on the afternoon when he looked up at me and yelled, "It never happened. I can't care. Put a dime in my head and the edges cut me, making slits in my mind."

His mind, indeed, is slit, although not still. His mind is dead but runs in frantic circles, so fast you can barely keep up.

"How are you doing today, Oscar?" I asked as I came into work one Monday morning. Oscar sat in the common room, face slick with sweat, eyes closed.

"Oh, my God," he said. He opened one eye, looked at me. "Oh, my God," he said again, jerking his fists into the air.

"It's OK, Oscar," I said. I sat down next to him. I knew what was coming, had seen it many times, but it never failed to unnerve me.

"It's OK," I said again. I wanted to put my hand on his shoulder, on the panicked pulse in his throat, but I was afraid he might confuse my touch with fire, with thorns.

"No no no no. It's success. I'm worried about my girls. My girls, Mikey took them. Can't for fire."

"There's no fire, Oscar. You're here, in the common room. I'm with you."

"Fire and my porn stars melting." He then did what he often did when upset, hurled himself backward against the wall and started to suckle his fingers, harder and harder, faster and faster. It didn't seem to soothe him this time. "Fire fire fire," he started to scream. "Isabella smells like semen. Get the sequins."

When Oscar has hallucinations, they are always about the same things, about porn stars in flames, porn stars with knives in their necks. Girls he has wanted to love come off as ash on the tips of his fingers.

"The Queen of England," he was saying now, his voice clipped in a mock British accent. "The Queen has stolen all my blow jobs." He stopped, pulled at his crotch, grunted. "Burning up, burning up, burning up!" Oscar resumed screaming now. His fists were jerking in the air. He slammed himself back into the couch, head pounding the wall.

"Sophie," I called. "Eddie."

But by the time they came to help, Oscar had gone mute again, eyes iced over, fists frozen in midair. Sophie looked at me, shrugged. Eddie walked out of the room. When I was alone with Oscar again, I did touch him. I pinched him lightly. No response. I reached out and tweaked his lower lip. No response. I raised my arm and slowly rested my hand on the crown of his head, right where the baby has the soft spot. I thought I could still feel it, the spongy flesh where the plates of bone had never grown, keeping him fetal and dreaming, always close to coma.

Six weeks ago, there was a late-night fire drill on the ward. In the past, drills have usually happened during the day and counselors have been allowed to escort patients from the building. But a new Massachusetts regulation now requires that no one receive help during a drill and that these drills also be sounded while patients are asleep, as a way of checking their response time and self-sufficiency during an emergency.

So in the middle of one night, a few months after Charles had died, the bells began to blare. Moxi, Robert, Lenny, Nick, all rose, clutching their blankets, pulling on robes, muttering as they went to stand on the sidewalk. The sky was clear, the dark air frosty. Ghosts rose from the mouths of the men. The night-shift counselors came out, took a head count, looked at their stopwatches. Very good, only three minutes, each demonstrating his mastery of what the Massachusetts Department of Mental Health calls "the self-preservation test."

"One . . . two . . . three," the counselors counted, checking each man off in their blue books. The men shivered, yawned, chuckled to themselves. But where was Oscar? "Five . . . six . . . seven," the counselors counted. "Eleven . . . twelve . . . thir—" No. Where was Oscar? They looked around.

Two-thirty A.M. in the inner city. The alarm still sounded, squawking into the night. Blue and red lights flashed from the ward windows. Far down the street an irritated neighbor yelled, "Shut the fuck up!" and one of the men whispered, "Up-shut-the-fuck-you," in response. Where was Oscar? At the end of the lawn, a bush moved in the breeze. Ed crept up to check it, thrashing at the branches with his flashlight. Oscar! Oscar? No Oscar. The men turned their heads left, now right. Some stared up at the moon.

"I'll go back in," Jen offered. She walked toward the red and blue lights. Up the ward's stairs she went, checking in the empty shower stall, the linen closet. The ward shook from the shrieking bells, and she muffed her ears with her hands.

She found Oscar, who, earlier that night had been alert and moving, lying comatose under his sheets. His face was pale and moist, his eyes half-shut shades, twin bars of blue between tiers of lashes. When she touched him, he didn't flinch, he was so far away. Did he hear the fire alarm and, terrified—with no one to help rouse him, guide him down the dark hallways that must, to him, flicker all the time with hallucinatory flames, patches of scorched skin—slip into a stupor? Or had he become catatonic for some other reason? We weren't sure.

"But if he can't pass the self-preservation test," Karen Conners, the assistant director, said the next day, "the state might not let him stay here, might ship him off to a more restrictive setting."

She called the Department of Mental Health and explained the problem to them. "Well," she said when she hung up the phone, "DMH says they've had this exact difficulty with a bunch of other patients on other wards, some who are heavily sedated, some just too out of it because of their psychosis. In any case"—and Karen chuckled—"they've designed a special electronic bed for these folks, to help them get moving on their own if there's a fire or a fire drill."

Six days later a large truck pulled up in front of our unit. The movers unloaded a bed, which they hauled up the stairs and exchanged for the one Oscar had been using. This bed was larger and bulkier, and beneath its mattress were coils of wires and strange red studs. The men drilled, hooked, and snapped, and within the hour the problem had been solved.

For this was a special bed, now connected to the fire alarm. When the alarm went off, the bed began to vibrate, sending deep, jerking pulses through the numbed skin of the psychotic. The vibrations weren't gentle—no tentative touches here, nothing slightly seductive like those cheap motel magic-finger mattresses. This bed could be more aptly called magic fists, for, on proper cue, it shook, seized, and bucked—a bronco bitten by a bee, impossible to stay on, impossible to sleep through; it was a bed to raise the dead, which was exactly what we needed.

We stood in the doorway to Oscar's room for a demonstration. Oscar wasn't home, had left the ward for day treatment. The alarm sounded; the mattress writhed, spasmed; discs hidden beneath its cotton covering rose and pummeled, then receded, only to rise again; I pictured Oscar in an ocean, his massive body made tiny by the hugeness of surrounding seas, a wave lifting him up by the fatty scruff of his neck, tossing him to the living shore. Surviving, after all. Opening his eyes to a blue sky and the grains of sand like glass in his open holes.

The state pays for men to stay on this ward for three to seven years. That makes sense to me, for seven years is the time it takes the body to slough off old cells and a new skin to form. Oscar, however, has been on this ward for nine years already and isn't getting well enough to go anywhere very soon.

He has seen men come and go, has witnessed graduations, deaths, the changing of staff. While he has been a patient here, two clinical directors have left to marry, and old counselors long moved on to other jobs have come back to visit with their babies. "Congratulations," Oscar muttered to his fellow patient Rich as Rich packed his bags, ready to leave after four years on the ward for a halfway house, a job. Oscar stood at the window, watched Rich trudge down the pathway, out onto the city street, a single suitcase in his hand.

"How do you feel about Rich moving on?" staff asked.

"Good for Rich," Oscar said, and turned away.

Staff believe Oscar is the most disconnected and delusional of the men on the ward. He talks only in grunts. He smokes four packs of cigarettes a day, and when he isn't doing that, he likes to lie in a corner. After a while, many men learn enough about the management of their mental illness that they can get a job in a sheltered workshop, but not Oscar, who, when he isn't chattering madly, stays in stiffened postures for hours or even days. "It's like I can't move," Oscar once said, trying to explain his catatonia to me. "I want to move but there are blockages everywhere. The air has holes and my muscles kill. I think even one step would slip me."

Another time he said, in a surprising burst of clearness, "I know I'm mentally ill but that doesn't mean I don't want to work someday. I do. I want to work in a garage with cars." He paused, with one finger probing his ear, then wiped the reddish wax on his pants. "Also," he said, "I would like someone to understand what's going on inside of me, why it's so hard for me to be alive-like." He looked up at the ceiling, tongued his teeth. "But instead," he continued, shaking his head, "I just talk more and more to myself."

And it's true, what Oscar says about how far he has swum from the world. While with the other men, staff have as a goal the eventual graduation or the achievement of part-time employment, with Oscar the most they hope for is that he master some very basic Activities of Daily Living skills. He needs to learn these things because his weight is so high, because he won't shower, and because almost every night he pees in his bed. Sometimes he defecates too. The ward smells of urine overlaid with Lysol. Each morning his soaked sheets are bundled into a ball and sent out to the cleaner. I wonder what the cleaner thinks when, every dawn, he receives these wet wrappings, too big to come from a baby's bed, smelling too strong for the body of the aged. The cleaner, I like to imagine, unwraps the sheets and rinses them, sprinkles them with powder that erupts into thousands of shimmery bubbles like beads of mercury shining. The bubbles move and froth, breathe light, break, and are born again. Far away, in his own stupor, with one leg raised rigidly in the air, Oscar feels the cleaner's hands massaging, the bubbles expanding, silky on his skin. He grins, giggles, a moment of comfort.

But the comforts are short-lived. "Jen," he says, coming into the office one morning early, just as we are beginning to meet. He stinks. He rubs one crusty eye with his fist. "Hi, everyone," he says, looking at the ceiling. "Jen, I got a problem."

"Yes, Oscar?"

Karen puts down her pencil and looks up. So do Eddie, Sophie, and I. "Well," he says, "I tried to wipe myself but couldn't get it all. Couldn't get it all. Couldn't get it—"

"Yes, Oscar?" Jen says again, more loudly. She's a young girl, just out of college, with fair skin and perfect, pouting lips.

Now Oscar comes right up to her, hefts himself close to her and repeats, "Couldn't get it all, couldn't get it all, know what I mean?"

Her fatal mistake is saying probably what all young psychology students are taught to say: "No, Oscar, what do you mean?"

"Well, I mean," he says, something edgy, compulsive in his voice, "I mean I couldn't get it all. Shit. I have shit on me, and it feels like pebbles. I couldn't get it all, see?" he says, and in one swift swipe he's pulling down his drawers, his enormous bare behind looming up. Jen shrinks backward.

"Oscar!" Karen says, stumbling forward, but Oscar is on a roll, on some kind of compulsive jag that psychologists call *perseverating*. "So when I sit," he says, "the cushion smells bad. It smells like dog."

Now Eddie is up too, and together Karen and he escort the bare-butted Oscar out of the office. Jen, Sophie, and I sit together, silent in the morning light. Jen's face is all wine and roses; her ears would be hot to the touch. "Oh, my God," Sophie says, and starts to laugh.

"Bare-assed Oscar, a nightmare vision," Jen says, and she starts to splutter too. But I think I see tears in her eyes—humiliation, fear.

"Yeah." I giggle along with them, but the giggles feel wrong, caught like bugs in my raw throat. We're all embarrassed, can't chase away from our minds the two looming moons of this man, the way he shoved his body into us, and in doing so brought us face-to-face with flesh. It's sometimes like that, working with the severely mentally ill. They force you into things you'd rather not see, not say. Oscar, with his fat and sweat and pee, brings us back to our own bodies. Right now, I simmer with shame.

And something else too. For lately, in the middle of the night, since I've known Oscar, since I've begun my work on this ward, I find myself startling awake. I think not only of Oscar in a swirl of craziness, but of Oscar in a stony stance. Eyes propped open. A fire alarm blaring and a man who cannot hear it. The streets in my own neighborhood are silent, and across the way I can see inside a neighbor's house, her win-

dow lit green with an aquarium, an underwater garden where anemones grow and open. I go toward the
aquarium, longing for the sleek pulse of fish, the
kinky wetness of seaweed. I wake up and can't feel
anything. Hysteria, I think. My arm is numb. My lips
are snow. I see Oscar glassed in, his madness dying
away to stillness. How even when he moves you cannot really reach him. I call to my boyfriend in the bed
next to me. *Make love to me,* I sometimes say. He
comes into me, but if I'm thinking of Oscar, it's sand
inside, grains of glass that hurt. It is nothing, a bone
sucked smooth as sleep.

This isn't the first time I've experienced bouts of
numbness. Ever since I was a little girl I've felt them
on and off, moments when the world drops away and
the possibility for connection dwindles. I go back to a
particular passage in one of Virginia Woolf's books,
where she talks about the jolt when the world recedes
and you see horror or you see nothing at all. Knowing
Oscar is knowing these moments again and again. It
is being brought back, first to shame, then to empti-
ness. It is a way of remembering, every time you see
that fat man's face, how not being is built into us as
certainly as is being. Every heartbeat has its opposite,
a snatching away of sound, an evaporation of blood.
Behind every presence lurks an absence. Loss, loss,
the animals cry.

. . .

I think, when all is said and done, that people prefer pain to nothingness. Maybe that's why all of us, especially the other men on the ward, have an easier time when Oscar is talking crazy than when he's catatonic. Because when Oscar is talking crazy, at least you know he's alive. He sweats and pees and sucks and shouts about fire, while at other times he's so still, so silent, like the highest animal cries that cannot be heard, living at a pitch too painful for human ears. At these times, Oscar crouches in the middle of the living room, one arm extended up into the air, or worse, he's on all fours in a rigid rigor mortis. I recall what he once said to me, how "it hurts to move because too much is happening. Too much comes in." Is catatonia a response not only to fear, but to an extreme sensitivity as well? Is Oscar aware, kneeling there, of the earth's slow rotation, a seismic shudder twitching under miles of muscular mass? Can he feel buried bones dissolving, a graveyard away a body being eaten by a beetle? Is he so much in touch that he's shed his psychic skin, the medium through which we absorb a livable world? The world isn't livable for Oscar.

And this makes the other patients angry. When he sits or stands in a stupor, they pace and mutter around him. A patient named Nick comes into the living room, kicks a comatose Oscar in the butt. "Wake up, you lunatic," he snarls. He stands there, arms crossed, waiting, and when he gets no response, he kicks him again. Then he leaves. "Can't watch any TV," he mutters, "because so long as that lunatic's there, it's all I'll see."

Silence does have a sound of its own, and the death pose, which is supposedly the body fading, is really its opposite, a florescence we cannot ignore. "Move, move," Robert wails, dancing around the dreaming Oscar, frantically probing him, now in the gut, now in the neck. Lenny comes in, creeps up. "Ahhh, Oscar," he keens. "Ahh, Oscar, disappear, disappear?" He extends one long finger, pulls back a puffy eyelid, stares in. I wonder if he sees himself, sees how far he can sink; I wonder if that's why he shudders, moves away. Joseph, obsessed with words, walks up to Oscar and angrily writes on him, pressing his pen hard into the piled flesh on his cheek, and what he writes is spidery, illegible, has a look of veins and webbing, a wish to bring the body back.

Only Moxi, who has made so much improvement in the past several months, seems to have the kind of quiet faith that allows Oscar to swim undisturbed through days of coma. I won't ever forget Moxi and how he comes up to Oscar, blows in the fat man's ear. Each time Oscar slips into a stupor, Moxi purses his lips and blows, sings softly in Vietnamese. Then he kneels down, lifts Oscar's shirt, and, taking the enormous belly between his two tan hands, presses his ear to the navel and listens. Moxi closes his eyes, smiles, every once in a while palpating the gut. I wonder if this is some sort of ancient Eastern healing ritual, or if Moxi, a man of deep belief, thinks there's a baby inside. "Something's inside," he whispers. "I must believe that. I won't forget her. A great wind. A heart."

"A great wind," I say to Oscar sometimes as I try to rouse him. "A heart." He doesn't move. He doesn't hear. She—we—are forgotten.

And then it's spring on the ward and the snow melts and the trees have a tender, wet look to them. The lawn outside turns a vivid green like some primitive dream, and when we peer out the windows we can almost imagine a snake among the blades. The men are restless. Joseph takes to scribbling senseless poems on the ward's walls, and Nick, before he goes out, dips into the bowl of condoms atop the TV, leaves with his pockets bulging.

The men clamor, complain about their dinners, the portions suddenly too small. Even Oscar joins in. "We don't want spaghetti," he announces in community meeting. "We want steak. Big bloody pieces of it."

We can't get steak, but pizza for sure. One warm May day seven of us—Moxi, Oscar, Lenny, Joseph, Nick, Robert, and I—trudge down the steep hill to the center of town. The men order single slices and cups of soda, except for Oscar. "Whole pie," he mutters to the counter help. He ambles over to the soda machine and slides quarter after quarter in, the machine belching back six, no seven, frosty bottles of pop.

We sit at the table and eat. Oscar scarfs, peels back the silver soda tabs, guzzles, and burps. "That's a sausage-smelling burp," Robert says, glowering.

Lenny holds his nose. "He'll pee for weeks," he says.

"Stink and stink," Nick chimes in.

Oscar appears not to have heard. His bloated eyelids flicker up, the whites foggy and distant. "Yeah," he says.

"You'll pee for weeks," Nick shouts, leaning close to Oscar as he guzzles. "And we all gotta smell it."

"Shhh," I say, looking around, glad that the pizza parlor is empty.

"Yeah," Oscar says. He takes a long stringy bite from a pepperoni piece, slurps up more soda.

"I hope at least you're enjoying your banquet, Oscar," I say.

Oscar suddenly puts down the crust he is munching. His mustache is clumped with chunks of tomato paste; a stray piece of pepperoni stays stuck to his chin. For a second his eyes focus, and when I turn around I see he's staring at his reflection in a pane of glass. "I'm not," he whispers. "I am not enjoying myself at all. I never have."

Something in the sound of his voice, its unusual clarity, makes the men stop, listen. The table gets quiet, our eyes all latched on to Oscar. Nick fiddles with his napkin; Robert shifts uncomfortably. "I can't taste a thing, you know," Oscar continues in this strange, sober soliloquy. He pauses, squints up at the ceiling, appears to be pondering his plight. "And it's because when I was two my father dropped me from a tree. He stole my taste buds, popping them off my tongue. Later on, I had an operation with a drill, before the fire. My body always buzzes. I can't feel nothing."

The table stays absolutely still. I look around at the men, but they don't move, mesmerized. I wonder if it's because they're simply surprised by Oscar's sudden clearness, or if he's doing more, speaking some larger sadness for them. And behind us the pizza man tosses a flabby wheel of dough, catches it with a soundless smack. Against the far wall a video-game screen flickers. Robotic miniature men, all mouths, devour one another, then blend back into blackness.

"I want outta here," Nick suddenly snarls. "I want outta this whole goddamn joint."

"Time to go," Lenny sings. He leaps up.

"Time to go," I echo dully, gathering paper plates and tossing them into the barrel.

Oscar, blank again, ambles out after us. We start our hike up the long hill, but a few feet into the climb Oscar abruptly stops, and I watch the rigidness ripple through his body, forcing his foot into stillness halfway out, tying his arms to his sides, cocking his head in a ridiculous posture. "Oscar," I nudge, "Oscar, Oscar."

The rest of the group pauses, looks back. "Oh, God," groans Nick. "Not a-fucking-gain."

"Come on, Oscar," I urge, my voice a little louder. "We have to head back now."

But Oscar, having just lapsed into a complete spell of stillness, hasn't heard, can't hear, his eyes lacquered with a thick glaze. Some people on the sidewalk stop, move cautiously around him. My mind ticks and reaches—how to hurl him from his stupor just long enough to get him home; how to propel him up this hill. And then, when I squint up the hill, I think I can suddenly see it from Oscar's perspective, a long steep snake you can't ever conquer, the pavement a painful rasp. Grass knifes up through the concrete cracks, where, right now, ants with wings devour their dead.

Who wouldn't want to distance themselves from such a vision? Who wouldn't want to weep? But we can't leave Oscar alone here. "All right," I say, catching my breath. I'm thinking of the nights when I startle awake, drawn toward the underwater garden, the aquarium, the beauty of bubbles floating up. "All right," I say to my group. "We're going to have to work together here. We can't leave Oscar like this in the middle of the street." And something in my own voice rises, sad. *Make love to me,* I say to my boyfriend, but sometimes not even that fleshy link can bring me back. What will bring Oscar back? The universe, astronomers say, is expanding out and out, but no galaxies fill the space. Only one tenth of the universe is packed with stars and suns; the other nine tenths lie in stuporous silence, utter, utter nothing.

"Everyone in back of Oscar," I say now. I feel my voice take on a sound at once pleading and strong. "And push."

"Get out of here," Nick says.

"Nick, get in here," I retort, and something edgy, even angry in my tone makes him listen.

The men gather behind Oscar, who is groaning softly to himself now. Moxi places his hands, with great precision, on the small of the back, Lenny on the shoulder blades, Robert on the buttocks. I look at the men and then—"Push!" I whoop. "Push!" Moxi whoops back. "Heave," Robert shouts. "Ho," Lenny answers.

And the men begin to edge this package of a person up the steep street. "Don't stop," Moxi puffs; "won't stop," Robert says; "heave," I cry; and then suddenly we're one mass moving together, pushing more than Oscar, pushing away the stupor that surrounds us all. I think of the men coming into the common room while Oscar stands stonily, how they probe him and beg him to resurrect himself. And now I watch the men's muscles flex, their faces drawn down in concentration, pointed with a purpose. There is something angry and loving in the way they force him forward. "Yes," chortles Joseph. "My man, my man," sings Lenny. Beads of sweat stand out on his black forehead.

"Exhale, inhale," I shout as we edge Oscar upward, and the men exhale together now, birthing this man, breathing Lamaze as, hands on his back, they urge his belly to open and spill a great wind, a heart.

We are covered with sweat by the time we've propelled a comatose Oscar to the top of the hill. "Staff," I yell as we stand outside the unit. Four daytime aides come down the path and lift Oscar up. "Thanks for the help," I say to the rest of the men, and they nod, drift off to the deck or the garden, where maybe they'll pull up grass by the roots, pressing the clean white wetness to their sweaty chins. Or pluck a new-formed crocus, staring into its center splashed with color, where right this minute a bee lowers its syringe, draws out pollen, food for the world.

And later on tonight, Oscar will wet the world. Lying in a daze in bed, eyes open and numbed, his body will release itself; his waters will break. And even though I know his major treatment goal is to conquer his incontinence, right now I hope, I really hope, he doesn't. What else can he do that's so real, so utterly warm and living? Why else am I drawn to the light of an aquarium at night? What other links do we have with our planet? For water, surely, is a link; water is the world's lubrication; the rivers are veins that feed flowers and bring together severed swatches of land.

And, leaning against the outside wall of the unit, I think about this. I think about the fact that some animals, when they have entered what scientists call the immobility response, can be roused with a strong spray. I close my eyes and envision a frozen Oscar, an Oscar too scared to move, now streaming, gushing, a rising river that douses his heated hallucinations and, clasping him, gives the silkiest of hugs. *Ssss* is the sound of Oscar's body singing at night. And I imagine Oscar on his own swollen creek. He paddles out of his room, down the ward hall, through the front door, and into the dark. Carried on his own current, he drifts back down that steep, impossible hill. He is easy movement now; he's immersed in the essence of things, for water is the essence of things, each drop made up of primeval matter, particles of hydrogen and oxygen that came together just as the earth was formed. And I, looking toward the lover I sometimes cannot reach, go with the floating Oscar. It's only in my mind, will always be only in my mind, and that's sad, but I can see it now, both of us lifted on yellow wave, creek wending its way to river, river to lake, lake swelling and merging with vast underwater gardens, the mouths of our seven seas; *sssss, bud, breathe,* and in this way joined, gently, with the rest of the moving world.

THREE SPHERES

Ms. Cogswell is a thirty-seven-year-old swf who has had over thirty hospitalizations, all for suicide attempts or self-mutilation. She scratches her arms lightly when upset. Was extensively sexually abused as a child. Is now requesting outpatient therapy for bulimia. Ms. Cogswell says she's vomiting multiple times during the day. Teeth are yellowed and rotting, probably due to stomach acids present during purges.

Client has been in outpatient therapy with over seventy (!) social workers, psychologists, and psychiatrists. She has "fired" them all because she cannot tolerate their limit-setting. She has threatened to sue "at least eight, maybe more," because "they never gave me what I needed. They were a menace to the profession." Please note: Client has never carried through with any of her threats to sue. She does, how-

*ever, demand complete access to her health-care
providers. Has a history of calling her therapists in
the middle of the night, screaming that she needs to
see them right away, and self-mutilating when her
requests are refused.*

*During her intake and evaluation appointment,
client presented as teary and soft-spoken. She wore
large hoop earrings and much makeup. She said she
believes she has gout and asked to be prescribed medication for it. Became belligerent when refused. Possibly this client is delusional, although she was fully
oriented to all three spheres—person, place, and
time—knowing who and where she was, and demonstrating capacity to locate historical figures in their
appropriate periods. Proverb interpretation: some-
what concrete. Serial sevens: intact. Recommenda-
tion: psychological testing; 1x weekly behavioral
therapy to address eating disorder; possible admission as an inpatient if she cannot get bulimia under
control.*

"So who wants to take the case?" asks Dr. Siley, the
director of both the inpatient and outpatient facilities
where I work. He folds the initial intake evaluation
from which he's been reading back into its green file.

None of the other clinicians offer. A woman as out-
rageously demanding and consistently suicidal as this

one is would add a lot of pressure to anyone's job. Ellen looks away. Veronica busies herself with the pleats on her skirt. The staff room stays quiet.

"What about you?" Dr. Siley says, looking in my direction. He knows my numbers are down. My job description states I'm responsible for seeing at least twenty in his outpatient clinic, in addition to the chronic schizophrenics in his residential program.

"Well," I say, "she sounds like a lot of work."

"Who isn't?" Veronica says.

"Why don't you take her, then?" I say.

"I'm full," Veronica says.

"And you aren't," Dr. Siley adds, pushing the file across the table toward me.

The phone rings six, maybe seven times, and then I hear a tiny voice on the other end—"Hello," it whispers, and I announce myself, the new therapist, let's make an appointment, look forward to meeting you, here's where the clinic is, in case you forgot—

"Can't," the voice weeps. "Can't, can't." I hear the sound of choking, the rustle of plastic. "Ten times a day," the voice says. "Into thirty-three gallon bags. I've spent"—and sobbing breaks out over the line— "I've spent every last penny on frozen pizzas. There's blood coming up now."

"You need to be in a hospital, then," I say.

"Oh, please," the voice cries. "Put me in a hospital before I kill myself. I'm afraid I'm going to kill myself."

I tell her to sit tight, hang on, and then I replace the receiver. I know the routine by heart. I call 911, give the ambulance company her name and address, tell them there's no need to commit her because she said she'd go willingly. Next they'll take her to an emergency room, and after that she'll be placed on an inpatient unit somewhere in the state. She can't come into our own program's inpatient unit because she's neither schizophrenic nor male, the two criteria for admission. She'll stay wherever she is put anywhere from three days to four weeks, enough time, probably, for her to forget I ever called, to forget she ever wandered into the clinic where I work. At the hospital they'll likely set her up with an aftercare psychologist affiliated with their own institution, and he or she will have to deal with what sounds like her enormous neediness. And I, lucky I, will be off the case. Or so I think.

Two days later a call comes through to my office. "Ms. Linda Cogswell tells us you're her outpatient therapist. Could you come in for a team meeting next Monday afternoon?"

"Well, I don't even know her, actually. I was assigned the case, but before I could meet her she had to be hospitalized. Where is she?"

"Mount Vernon. I'm her attending psychologist here. Would you be willing to meet with us regarding her aftercare plans?"

Mount Vernon, Mount Vernon. And suddenly, even though it's been years, I see the place perfectly all over again, the brick buildings, the green ivy swarming the windows. The nurses who floated down the halls like flocks of seagulls, carrying needles in their beaks. My heart quickens; a screw tightens in my throat.

"Mount Vernon?" I say. Of all the hundreds of hospitals in Massachusetts, why did it have to be *this* one? And another part of me thinks I should have been prepared, for eventually past meets present; ghosts slither through all sealed spaces.

"Look, I don't know the woman at all," I repeat, and I hear something desperate in my voice. I try to tamp it down, assume a professional pose. "I mean, the patient, although technically assigned to me, has not begun a formal course of psychotherapy under my care."

A pause on the line. "But *technically*," the voice retorts, "she is under your care, yes? You have some sort of record on her? Your clinic agreed to take the case?"

"Yes," I say. "Well . . . yes."

"Next Monday, then, one o'clock, North—"

"Two," I interrupt bitterly. "North Two."

"Good," she says. "We'll see you then."

What else can I do? Technically, I *have* been assigned the case. But this isn't any longer about the case; my hesitations now don't have to do with Linda Cogswell and her stained teeth, but with ivy on the brick, the shadow of a nurse, a needle, the way night looked as it fell beyond the bars and the stars were sliced into even segments. I remember looking out the windows on North Two; I remember Rosemary swallowing her hidden pills, how she danced the Demerol onto her tongue and later sank into a sleep so deep only the slamming cuffs of a cardiac machine could rouse her. Liquid crimson medicines were served in plastic cups. The rooms had no mirrors.

But the reflections came clear to me then, come still in quiet moments when past meets present so smoothly the seams disappear and time itself turns fluid. Sometimes I wish time stayed solid, in separable chunks as distinct as the sound of the ticking clock on my mantel. In truth, though, we break all boundaries, hurtling forward through hope and backward on the trail made by memory.

But what else can we do except reach, except remember? What else can I do, having been assigned this case? I will go in, go down. Go back.

American culture abounds with marketplace confessions. I know this. And I know the criticisms levied against this trend, how such open testifying trivializes suffering and contributes to the narcissism polluting our country's character. I agree with some of what the critics of the confessional claim. I'm well aware of Wendy Kaminer's deep and, in part, justified scorn for the open admissions of Kitty Dukakis, who parades her alcoholism for all to observe, or for Oprah, who extracts admissions from the soul like a dentist pulls teeth, gleefully waving the bloodied root and probing the hole in the abscessed gum while all look, without shame, into the mouth of pain made ridiculously public. Would it not be more prudent to say little or nothing, to hold myself back like any good doctor, at most admitting some kind of empathic twinge? For what purpose will I show myself? Does it satisfy some narcissistic need in me—at last I can have some of the spotlight? Perhaps a bit, yes? But I think I set aspects of my own life down not so much to revel in their gothic qualities, but to tell you this: that with many of my patients I feel intimacy, I feel love. To say I believe time is fluid, and so are the boundaries between human beings, the border separating helper from the one who hurts always blurry. Wounds, I think, are never confined to a single skin but reach out to rasp us all. When you die, there's that much less breath to the world, and across continents someone supposedly separate gasps for air. When, Marie, Joseph, Peter,

Moxi, Oscar, when I weep for you, don't forget I weep as well for me.

I have to drive out of the city to get there, down forty miles of roads I've avoided for the past eight years. Where there was once farmland, horses spitting sand as they galloped, wide willow trees I sat under when the nurses let me out on passes, there are now squat, square houses dotting the hills. But the building's bubbled dome rises unmistakably over a crest as I round the corner, floating there in the distance like a glittering spaceship, looking exactly the same as it did almost a decade ago. Walking back from passes, I would see that domed bubble, that silver blister bursting against a spring sky, and I would count, *One* . . . *two* . . . *three* . . . getting closer, my heart hammering half with fear, half with relief. Safe again. Trapped again. Safe again. Trapped aga—

And I have the same heart in the same socket of chest, and it hammers the way it used to, and I find myself thinking the same words, *Safe again, trapped again.* My palms sweat on the steering wheel. I remind myself: I am *not* that girl. I am *not* that girl. I've changed. I've grown. It's a long time ago. I am now a psychologist, who over the year has learned to give up her Indian-print sundresses and bulky smocks for tailored skirts, who carries a black Coach leather briefcase. How often, though, I've marveled at the discrepancy between this current image of me and the tangled past it sprang from. Sometimes I've imagined shouting out in staff meeting, in front of all my colleagues, who know me as a spunky confident doctor, how often I've wanted to say, *Once I, too*—

And what I would tell them goes something like this. On five separate occasions, spanning the ages from fourteen to twenty-four, I spent considerable portions of my life inside the very hospital whose graveled drive I am now turning into. Until what could be called my "recovery" at twenty-five or so, I was admitted to this institution on the average of every other year for up to several months. And even today, at thirty-one years old, with all of that supposedly behind me, with chunks of time in which to construct and explain the problems that led me to lockup, I find myself at a loss for words. Images come, and perhaps in the images I can illuminate some of my story. I am ten years old, sitting under the piano, as my mother, her face a mask of pain, pummels the keys. Beneath the bench I press the golden pedals, hold them all down at the same time so our house swells with raw and echoing sounds, with crashing crescendos and wails that shiver up inside my skin, lodging there a fear of a world I know is impossible to negotiate, teetering on a cruel and warbling axis. And later, while I am lying in my bed, she murmurs a Hebrew prayer and I imagine her hands exploring me, and a darkness sprouts inside my stomach. A pain grows like a plant, and when I was twelve, thirteen, I decided to find the plant, grasping for its roots with a razor blade. Stocked solid with the romance of the teenage years, with the words of the wounded Hamlet and the drowned Virginia Woolf, whom I adored, I pranced on the lawn of my school, showing off the fresh gashes—Cordelia, a dwarf, a clown, Miss Havisham. I loved it all. I wept for the things inserted into me, the things plucked out of me. And I knew, with the conviction of adolescence, that pain confers a crown. I was removed to the hospital, then a foster home, then the hospital, again and again. Later on, in my late teens and early twenties, I starved myself, took pills to calm myself down, wanted a way out. And finally I found one, or one, perhaps, found me.

I am not that girl any longer. I tell that to myself as I ride up the hospital's elevator. I found some sort of way into recovery. But I know, have always known, that I could go back. Mysterious neurons collide and break. The brain bruises. Memories you thought were buried rise up.

I rise up in the elevator and the doors part with a whisper. Stepping off, I find myself face-to-face with yet another door, this one bolted and on it a sign that says: ENTER WITH CAUTION. SPLIT RISK.

And now I am standing on the other side of that door—the wrong, I mean the right, side of the door, and I ring the buzzer. I look through the thick glass window and see a nurse hustle down the hall, clipboard in hand. I recognize her. Oh, my God, I recognize her! I hunch, dart back. Impossible, I tell myself. It's been over eight years. Staff turnover in these places is unbelievably high. But it could be her, couldn't it? And what happens if she recognizes me? My mouth dries and something shrivels in my throat.

"Dr. Slater?" she asks, opening the door. I nod, peer into her eyes. They're the blue of sadness, thickly fringed. Her lips are painted the palest sheen of pink. "Welcome," she says, and she steps back to let me pass. I was wrong—I've never seen this woman in my life. I don't know those eyes, their liquid color, nor the voice, in whose tone I hear, to my surprise, a ring of deference. Doctor—she actually calls me doctor. She bends a bit at the waist, in greeting, acknowledging the hierarchies that exist in these places—nurses below psychologists, psychologists below psychiatrists, patients at the bottom of the ladder.

With a sudden surge of confidence, I step through. The reversal is remarkable, and for a second it makes me giddy. I'm aware of the incredible elasticity of life, how the buckled can become straight, the broken mended. Watch what is on the ground; watch what you step on, for it could contain hidden powers and, in a rage, fly up all emerald and scarlet to sting your face.

And here I am, for the briefest moment, all emerald, all scarlet. "Get me a glass of water," I imagine barking to her. "Take your pills or I'll put you in the quiet room."

Then the particular kind of dense quiet that sits over the ward comes to me. Emerald goes. Scarlet dies down. I am me again, here again. I grip my briefcase and look down the shadowy hall, and it's the same shadowy hall, loaded with the exact same scents, as it was so many years ago. The paint is that precise golden green. The odor is still undefinable, sweet and wretched. Another woman comes up, shakes my hand. "I'm Nancy," she says, "charge nurse on the unit."

"Good to meet you," I say. And then I think I see her squint at me. I've the urge to toss my hair in front of my face, to mention a childhood in California or Europe, how I've only been in this state for a year.

"We're meeting in the conference room," Nancy says. Clutching my briefcase, I follow her down the corridor. We pass open doors, and I hold my breath as we come to the one numbered 6, because that was my bedroom for many of the months I stayed here. I slow down, try to peer in. Just as they used to, heavy curtains hang over a large, thickly meshed window. *There are the stars,* I want to say, for in my mind it's night again, and someone is rocking in a corner. Now, in the present time, a blond woman lies in what used to be my bed. On that mattress swim my cells, the ones we slough off, the pieces of ourselves we leave behind, forever setting our signatures into the skin of the world. As she sleeps, my name etches itself on her smooth flesh, and my old pain pours into her head.

And just as we are passing her by, the woman leaps out of bed and gallops to the door. "Oh, Nancy," she keens. "I'm not safe, not safe. Get my doctor. I want my doctor."

"Dr. Ness will be up to see you at four," Nancy says.

Suddenly the woman snarls, "Four. Dr. Ness is always late. Always keeps me waiting. I want a new doctor, someone who'll really care. A new doctor, a new—"

Her voice rises and she sucks on her fist. "Stop it, Kayla," Nancy says. "Take your fist out of your mouth. You're twenty-nine years old. And if you want a new doctor, you'll have to bring it up in community meeting."

Kayla stamps her foot, tosses her head like a regal pony. "Screw you," she mutters now. "Screw this whole fucking place," and then she stomps back into her bed.

When we're a few feet beyond the scene, Nancy turns to me, smiles conspiratorially. I feel my mouth stretched into a similar smirk, and it relieves yet bothers me, this expression toward a patient. "Borderline," Nancy says matter-of-factly, giving a crisp nod of her head.

I sigh and nod back. "They're exhausting patients, the ones with borderline personalities." I pause. "But I prefer them to antisocials," I add, and as I say these words I feel safe again, hidden behind my professional mask. I am back on balance, tossing jargon with the confidence of a Brahman in a village of untouchables. There is betrayal here, in what I do, but in betrayal I am finally camouflaged.

Of all the psychiatric illnesses, borderline personality disorder may be the one professionals most dislike to encounter. It's less serious than, say, schizophrenia, for the borderline isn't usually psychotic, but such patients are known for their flamboyant, attention-getting, over-demanding ways of relating to others.

Linda, according to her intake description, is surely a borderline. Patients like her are described with such adjectives as "manipulative" and "needy," and their behaviors are usually terribly destructive and include anorexia, substance abuse, self-mutilation, suicide attempts. Borderlines are thought to be pretty hopeless, supposedly never maturing from their "lifelong" condition. I myself was diagnosed with, among other things, borderline personality disorder. In fact, when I left the hospital for what I somehow knew would be the very last time, at twenty-four years old, I asked for a copy of my chart, which is every patient's right. The initial intake evaluation looked quite similar to Linda's, and the write-ups were full of all kinds of hopeless projections. "This young woman displays a long history marked by instability in her interpersonal and intrapsychic functioning," my record read. "She clearly has had a long career as a mental patient and we will likely encounter her as an admission again in the future."

I recall these words now, as we enter the conference room, where several other nurses and doctors sit around a table with a one-way mirror on the far wall. I scan their faces quickly, praying I look as unfamiliar to them as they do to me. I don't recognize any of the people in here, and I'm hoping against hope they don't recognize me. Still, even if we've never met, I feel I know them somehow, know them in a deep and private part of me. "Ta da," I have the angry urge to shout out, bowing to the bearded psychiatrist at the oval's head, standing arms akimbo, twirling so my skirt swells out. "Here I am," I'd like to yell. "Yes, sireee, encountered again. Guess who you're looking at; guess who this is. The Borderline! And sure enough, folks, I *did* mature out, at least a little . . ."

Of course I won't say such a thing, wouldn't dare, for I would lose my credibility. But the funny thing is, I'm supposedly in a profession that values honesty and self-revelation. Freud himself claimed you couldn't do good analytic work until you'd "come clean" with yourself in the presence of another, until you'd spoken in the bright daylight your repressed secrets and memories. Freud told us not to be so ashamed, to set loose and let waltz our mothers and fathers, our wetness and skins. Training programs for psychologists like me, and the clinics we later work in, have as a credo the admission and discussion of countertransference, which by necessity claims elements of private conflict.

But at the same time, another, more subtle yet powerful message gets transmitted to practitioners in the field. This message says, *Admit your pain, but only to a point. Admit it but keep it clean. Go into therapy, but don't call yourself one of us if you're* anything *more than nicely neurotic.* The field transmits this message by perpetuating so strongly an us-versus-them mindset, by consistently placing a rift between practitioners and patients, a rift it intends to keep deep. This rift is reflected in the language only practitioners are privy to, in words like *glossolalia* and *echolalia* instead of just saying *the music of madness,* and then again in phrases like *homicidal ideation* and *oriented to all three spheres* instead of *he's so mad he wants to kill her* or *he's thinking clearly today, knows who, what, and where he is.* Along these same lines, practitioners are allowed to admit their *countertransference* but not the *pain pain pain the patient brings me back to, memories of when I was five, your arms, my arms, and the wound is one.* No. To speak in such a way would make the rift disappear, and practitioners might sink into something overwhelming. We—I—hang on to the jargon that at once describes suffering and hoists us above it. Suddenly, however, here I am, back in an old home, lowered.

I recognize the conference room as the place where, when I was fourteen, I met with my mother and the social worker for the last time. My father had gone away to Egypt. My mother, abandoned by him, somehow always abandoned and lonely, even as she surrounded herself with people, was wearing a scarf around her neck and a gold Star of David wedged between the hills of her breasts. Years later, seeing the mountains of Jerusalem, cupping the scathing sand of the desert, hearing the primitive wails of the Hasids who mourned the Temple's destruction, I would think of my mother's burning body, a pain I could never comprehend.

This is the conference room where she, unstable, rageful, maybe delusional at times, shot through with a perpetual anxiety that made her hands shake, told me she was giving me up, giving me over to become a foster child. "I can't handle you anymore," she'd said to me, spit at me. "I no longer want you in my house."

I bow my head in deference to something I cannot name, and enter the room. Things are screaming inside me and my eyes feel hot. Nancy introduces me all around, and I take a seat, pull out a notebook, try to act as calm and composed as possible. "The patient Ms. Cogswell," the bearded psychiatrist begins, "is not able to make good use of the hospital. She's an extreme borderline, wreaking havoc on the unit. We suspect her of some factitious posturing as well." He pauses, looks at me, clears his throat. I smile back at him but my mouth feels uncoordinated, tightness at its corners. I won't cry, won't cry, even though in the one-way mirror, in the criss-crossing of the creamy branches beyond the ward's windows, I see my mother again, her face coming to me clearly, her eyes haunted with loneliness and rage. I feel her fingers at my breasts and flinch.

"We think," a social worker named Miss Norton continues, "that we'll be discharging her in a matter of days, as soon as we get her stabilized on some meds. We take it you'll be picking up her case on an outpatient basis. Any ideas of how you'll work with her?"

I nod, pretend to make some notes on the pad. As my voice rises through my throat, I'm surprised at how smooth it sounds, a sleek bolt of silk. "Lots of limits," I say. "We know borderlines do well with lots of limits. This is the only context in which a workable transference can begin."

The bearded doctor nods. In the tree, my mother tongues her teeth and wind lifts her lovely skirt, embroidered with fragile flowers. And then she is not my mother anymore, but a little girl whose legs are white, a single ruby scar on scrubbed knee. And while part of me sits in the conference room, part of me flies out to meet this girl, to touch the sore spot, fondling it with my fingers.

For I have learned how to soothe the hot spots, how to salve the soreness on my skin. I can do it so no one notices, can do it while I teach a class if I need to, or lead a seminar on psychodiagnosis. I can do it while I talk to you in the evenest of tones. "Shhhh," I whisper to the hurting part, hidden here. You can call her borderline—call me borderline—or multiple, or heaped with posttraumatic stress—but strip away the language and you find something simple. You find me, part healthy as a horse and part still suffering, as are we all. What sets me apart from Kayla or Linda or my other patients like Oscar, Marie, Moxi—what sets me apart from these "sick" ones—is simply a learned ability to manage the blades of deep pain with a little bit of dexterity. Mental health doesn't mean making the pains go away. I don't believe they ever go away. I do believe that nearly every person sitting at this oval table now has the same warped impulses, the same scarlet id, as the wobbliest of borderlines, the most florid of psychotics. Only the muscles to hold things in check—to channel and funnel—are stronger. I have not healed so much as learned to sit still and wait while pain does its dancing work, trying not to panic or twist in ways that make the blades tear deeper, finally infecting the wounds.

Still, I wonder. Why—how—have I managed to learn these things while others have not? Why have I managed somehow to leave behind at least for now what looks like wreckage, and shape something solid from my life? My prognosis, after all, was very poor. In idle moments, I still slide my fingers under the sleeves of my shirt and trace the raised white nubs of scars that track my arms from years and years of cutting. How did I learn to stop cutting and collapsing, and can I somehow transmit this ability to others? I don't know. It's a core question for me in my work. I believe my strength has something to do with memory, with that concept of fluid time. For while I recall with clarity the terror of abuse, I also recall the green and lovely dream of childhood, the moist membrane of a leaf against my nose, the toads that peed a golden pool in the palm of my hand. Pleasures, pleasures, the recollections of which have injected me with a firm and unshakable faith. I believe Dostoevski when he wrote, "If one has only one good memory left in one's heart, even that may be the means of saving us." I have gone by memory.

And other things too. E. J. Anthony wrote in his landmark study, *The Invulnerable Child*, that some children manage to avoid or grow out of traumatic pasts when there is the presence in their lives of at least one stable adult—an aunt, a neighbor, a teacher. I had the extreme good fortune to be placed in a foster home where I stayed for four years, until I turned eighteen, where I was lovingly cared about and believed in. Even when my behavior was so bad I cut myself in their kitchen with the steak knife, or when, out of rage, I swallowed all the Excedrin in their medicine cabinet and had to go back to the unit, my foster parents continued to believe in my abilities to grow, and showed this belief by accepting me after each hospital discharge as their foster child still. That steady acceptance must have had an impact, teaching me slowly over the years how to see something salvageable in myself. Bless those people, for they are a part of my faith's firmness. Bless the stories my foster mother read to me, the stories of mine she later listened to, her thin blond hair hanging down in a single sheet. The house, old and shingled, with niches and culverts I loved to crawl in, where the rain pinged on a leaky roof and out in the puddled yard a beautiful German shepherd, who licked my face and offered me his paw, barked and played in the water. Bless the night there, the hallway light they left on for me, burning a soft yellow wedge that I turned into a wing, a woman, an entire army of angels who, I learned to imagine, knew just how to sing me to sleep.

At a break in the conference, a nurse offers me a cup of coffee. "Sure," I say, "but first the ladies' room." And then I'm off, striding down the hallway I know so well, its twists and turns etched in subterranean memory. I go left, then right, swing open the old wooden ladies' room door, and sit in a stall.

When I come back, the nurse is ready with a steaming plastic cup. She looks at me, puzzled, as she hands me my hot coffee. "You've been here before?" she asks.

My face must show some surprise, for she adds, "I mean, the bathrooms. You know where they are."

"Oh," I say quickly. "Right. I've visited some of my patients on this ward before, yes."

"You don't have to use the patient bathroom," she says, smiling oddly, looking at me with what I think may be suspicion. "We don't recommend it," she adds. "Please use the staff bathroom, through the nurse's station."

"OK," I say. I bend my face into the coffee's steam, hoping she'll think the redness is from the rising heat. Of course. How stupid of me. What's she thinking? Can she guess? But in a way I *am* one of the patients, and she could be too. I'm not ready to say it yet, though. Weak one. Wise one. This time, memory has led me astray.

The conference resumes. I pay little attention. I'm thinking about the faux pas with the bathroom, and then I'm watching the wind in the tree outside the window. I am thinking about how we all share a similar, if not single pain, and the rifts between stalls and selves is its own form of delusion. And then I hear, through a thin ceiling, wails twining down, a sharp scream, the clattering of footsteps. I sit up straight.

"Delivery room," the social worker says, pointing up. "We're one floor under the maternity ward."

I smile. That's right. North Two is just one floor of what is an old large public hospital. The psychiatric unit we're on has always been wedged between labor rooms upstairs and a nursery downstairs. When I was a patient, I could often hear, during group therapy or as I drifted into a drugged sleep, the cries of pushing women as their muscles contracted and in great pain their pink skins ripped, a head coming to crown.

"Why don't you meet with Linda now," the psychiatrist says, checking his watch and gathering his papers. Everyone stands, signaling the end of the conference.

"You can take one of the interview rooms," Nancy, the charge nurse, adds. "They're nice places for doing therapy, comfortable."

I nod. I've almost forgotten about Linda and how she is the reason for my return here today. Now I walk with the rest out of the conference room and Nancy points down the long hall. "There," she says, her finger aiming toward a door on the left. "The third room. We'll bring Linda to you." And then, to my surprise, Nancy fishes deep into her pocket and pulls out a large steel ring of keys, placing them in my hand. They're the same keys, I know, from all those years ago, keys I was not allowed to touch but that I watched avidly whenever I could, the cold green gleam and mysterious squared prongs opening doors to worlds I didn't know how to get to. Keys, keys, they are what every mental patient must dream of, the heart-shaped holes keys fit into, the smart click as they twist the secret tumblers and unlatch boxes, velvet-lined and studded with sea jewels. Keys are symbols of freedom and power and finally separateness. For in a mental hospital, only one side has the keys; the others go to meals with plastic forks in their fists.

Slowly, I make my way down the hall to the interview room, stand outside the locked door holding the key ring. It feels cool, and I press it to my cheek. A hand there once, feeling me for a fever, stroking away my fear. Bless those who have helped.

A woman who looks far older than her thirty-seven years is now making her way down the hall. Stooped, she is, with tired red ringlets of hair. As she gets closer I see the dark ditches under her eyes, where years of fatigue and fear have gathered. I would like to put my finger there, sweep away the microscopic detritus of suffering.

"Linda," I say, and as she comes close to me, I extend my hand. "Hello," I say, and I can hear a gentleness in my voice, a warm wind in me, for I am greeting not only her, but myself.

We stand in front of the locked interview room and I fumble for the correct key. I start to insert it in the lock, but then, halfway done, I stop. "You," I say to my new patient, Linda. "You take the key. You turn the lock."

She arches one eyebrow, stares up at me. Her face seems to say, *Who are you, anyway?* I want to cry. The hours here have been too long and hard. "You," I say again, and then I feel my eyes actually begin to tear. She steps forward, peers closely, her expression confused. Surely she's never seen one of her doctors cry. "It's OK," I say. "I know what I'm doing." And for a reason I cannot quite articulate at the moment, I make no effort to hide the wetness. I look straight at her. At the same time, for the first time today, my voice feels genuinely confident. "Take the keys, Linda," I say, "and open the door."

She reaches out a bony hand, takes the keys from me, and swings open the door. The interview room is shining with sun, one wall all windows. I've been in this room too, probably hundreds of times over the years, meeting with the psychiatrists who tried to treat me. I shiver with the memory. Ultimately it was not their treatments or their theories that helped me get better, but the kindness lodged in a difficult world. And from the floor above comes the cry of a protesting baby, a woman ripped raw in birth. She is us. We are her. As my mother used to say, rocking over the Shabbat candles, chanting Jewish prayers late, late into the night, "Hear, O Israel. The Lord our God, the Lord is one, and so are we as a people."

She would pause then, her hands held cupped over the candlesticks. "We are one," she would repeat to me after a few moments, her strained face peering at me through shadows. "As a people we are always one."

Sometimes I miss her.

My patient and I sit down, look at each other. I see myself in her. I trust she sees herself in me.

This is where we begin.